For Krishna, my wife, my love, my best friend,

who is battling this insidious disease …..

Copyright © 2020 JGM Alexander

revised edition 2021

All rights reserved

Cover design by Lekha Nanavati

Acknowledgements

I would like to thank the staff of the NHS in Scotland who have given my wife endless support. It truly is an exemplary organisation staffed with the most dedicated of individuals.

Also, thank you to Ms. Shilpa Sapat for her insight and useful suggestions.

In addition, we would like to thank our doctor in Italy, Dott. Francesca Michelucci in Pisa, who has guided us through the Coimbra protocol and provided support and encouragement when we have hit the inevitable bumps in the road.

Contents

Acknowledgements ii
Table of Figures 4
1. Introduction 5
2. The First Signs & Diagnosis 10
    Denial 11
    Hillwalking 14
    Dizziness 15
    Weakness 16
3. The Treatment 18
    Side Effects and Risks 19
    Exploring Alternatives 21
4. The Basis of Science 24
    The Scientific Method 24
    The Growth of Pharmaceuticals 28
    Behaviour and Ethics 30
    Vitamins 32
    The Rise of Additives 35
    Evolution of the Medical Practitioner 38
5. The Influence of Timing 43
    First Indications 43

Multiple Sclerosis Types 46

Optimistic Time? 51

6. A New Hope 52

The Jelinek Approach 53

Our Adoption of Jelinek's Methodology 73

7. The Immune System 77

The Innate Immune System 79

The Adaptive Immune System 81

T and B Cells and MS 92

Other Things to Consider 97

Gedankenexperiment 99

8. The Bumpy Road 105

Ayurvedic Treatments 105

Introduction to the Coimbra Protocol 109

The Treatments 113

Our Actual Journey 115

Hypercalcemia 118

Reviewing the Protocol 120

9. Improving Behaviour 123

Twenty Questions 123

Cognition 125

Don't Make Assumptions 126

Patience	127
Tactful Risk Management	129
Not Rock Hudson, James Bond	132
10. Final Discussion	134
Root Cause	134
Now What?	138
Being a Better Partner	139
Finally	140
References	142
About the Author	150

Table of Figures

FIGURE 1 : SARA CURVE 12

FIGURE 2 : RRMS PROGRESSION 48

FIGURE 3 : PPMS PROGRESSION 49

FIGURE 4 : SPMS PROGRESSION 50

FIGURE 5 : MS FAT CONSUMPTION BY COUNTRY 57

FIGURE 6 : MS MORTALITY BY COUNTRY 60

FIGURE 7 : VITAMIN D3 PRODUCTION 61

FIGURE 8 : B CELL DIFFERENTIATION 82

FIGURE 9 : T CELL ACTIVATION (1) 88

FIGURE 10 : T CELL ACTIVATION (2) 89

FIGURE 11 : T CELL ACTIVATION (3) 90

FIGURE 12 : TH17 AND T REG BALANCE 94

FIGURE 13 : DAMAGED NERVE BY T CELL ATTACK 100

FIGURE 14 : REDUCTION IN RELAPSES WITH D3 109

FIGURE 15 : PTH MEASURE 2017-18 116

FIGURE 16 : PTH MEASURE 2018-19 118

FIGURE 17: TRACKING KIDNEY FUNCTION 121

1. Introduction

"If there's a book that you want to read, but it hasn't been written yet, then you must write it." This is a quote from Toni Morrison, the Nobel Laureate who died in 2019, and it helped inspire me to write what follows.

There are a lot of self-help books for Multiple Sclerosis sufferers. However, I could not find one that was written from a partner's point of view. So, I wanted to tell you our story, that is, of my wife, who has Relapsing Remitting Multiple Sclerosis (RRMS) and myself, who does not, but who, over the past few years, it would be fair to say, has suffered from an increased level of anxiety.

I'll take you through our journey from initial signs, which we dismissed, to the reality of the diagnosis. Our emotional low points, and our determination to fight this insidious disease. I shall also endeavour to be honest about myself, as to how annoying a partner can be. The odd reality is that the affected patient seems to be more sanguine about the prognosis. The powerless partner, who has no direct information regarding how well the MS patient is feeling, is left in a state of limbo without any means or understanding about what the best course of action should be taken.

I recall a 1950's Hollywood melodrama called 'Magnificent Obsession'. Basically, the plot is spoiled playboy, Rock Hudson, through a series of events falls for the wife of the doctor who had died. Unfortunately, he then manages to run her down in a car and cause her blindness. Apparently, there was no cure possible, so Rock Hudson dedicates himself to become a brain surgeon. Some years later he seeks her out, performs an operation, she then awakes, and can see!

I am not, by any stretch of the imagination, recommending this film. However, I do feel that one should never give up and that there are always possibilities. As I said, I want to take you through our journey. As you will find out this included a significant amount of research. I do not believe that I am Rock Hudson, however, as I shall discuss later, there is a lot of evidence in published literature that can point to some interventions that may help. I include it so that you can make up your own minds regarding available courses of action.

Everyone knows that MS was not well understood, and in particular the root cause. The mechanism that initiated the disease was unknown. In fact, one of the first doctors that we saw reminisced that when he was a medical student it was thought to be caused by radiation from the granite in Aberdeen!

The good news, such that it is, is that the understanding has come a long way since then.

It's probably worth giving a little background about myself which may help clarify how I fit into the story. From my childhood my interests were science. Initially, astronomy and then physics. I was fortunate to study physics as an undergraduate and then research into ship dynamics as a post-graduate. Now, to be fair, none of this is remotely connected to medicine, bioscience or pharmacology, so you will be wondering how I could possibly support my wife's journey in anything more than providing emotional sustenance. I do, however, have the ability to read, digest information and draw logical conclusions. My wife thinks, probably rightly, that I can be a bit obsessive if I have a problem to solve. I also have a stubborn streak and a fundamental belief in cause and effect, even if it's not obvious what may be the root cause.

I do not have the resources to undertake research into MS, however, as I have said there is a lot of information out there. With time it is possible to build a picture of potential influencing factors that impact MS, and at the very least take steps to avoid or minimise these. One thing that is important is to remember that all research must be viewed with a critical eye. The basis of proof is to ensure experimental repeatability.

So, given the above, and the desire to share the problem and not just sit in the corner helplessly waiting on whatever fate has in store for us, I set about to read and understand as much as I could. Not to make some miraculous breakthrough. After all, I'm not Rock Hudson! It was really about becoming empowered to question whatever treatments were offered, or at least question why treatments were not offered. At least, that's how it began. As I read more, I was surprised to find out that some of the practices in the industry and in the numerous self-help guides were, to say the least, questionable, disingenuous or maybe even dangerous.

As I tried to build up an understanding of the mechanisms at play, I by necessity, had to read a number of academic papers. I have provided references for anyone inclined to follow the logic that led to our journey. Just to be clear, there are many paths that may be followed. This is just one, that has, to date, suited us, but one based on as much evidence as I could find.

In the subsequent chapters I shall describe the journey my wife and I have been on during the last few years, the ups and downs, the hope and the despair, and the focus that I needed to stop me feeling useless and eunuch like.

2. The First Signs & Diagnosis

Hindsight is fantastic. It makes us all experts. It's the twenty-twenty vision on the past. Unfortunately, as we progress through life, making a judgement about the facts presented before us in real time can be a lot more problematic. Unless you are actively looking for them, clues can be, and often are, missed. Only with hindsight can a pattern be established. Fairly innocuous symptoms that are easily dismissed could be the first signs of something more insidious.

In the early 2000's my wife would wake up saying that she had pins and needles in her legs. We usually put this down to sleeping in an odd position, and as the sensation did not last long and there seemed to be no ill effects, it was dismissed. After some time, the sensation stopped recurring. I cannot recall how long this went on for, but I'm sure that it was reasonably short lived. Now, I cannot say whether this was an early indicator of MS, but it cannot be dismissed. Needless to say, we did nothing, and life carried on as usual.

The first serious sign that something was amiss was when she suddenly developed a blurriness in one eye. Again, with no experience of any autoimmune disease our thoughts were along the line of an eye infection.

However, the optician referred us to the local doctor who suggested an MRI scan. In our naivety we had no idea of the path we were being led down.

The reality was that this event was, in all likelihood, the Clinically Isolated Syndrome (CIS, see chapter 5). If we had known the implications of such an occurrence, then our judgement of the diagnosis may have been significantly different.

The medical teaching hospitals are second to none. They have a well-established reputation and lead the world in many fields. However, one of the down sides is that medical students and young doctors have to learn. The doctor that my wife saw clearly knew the demographic for MS in Scotland (~209 cases per 100000), therefore, for a woman in her mid 30s with an obvious indicator as eye blurriness, then MS must be considered as a possible contender. Thus, the news was broken that this was likely to be MS!

Denial

Any psychologist will tell you that there is a standard response pattern to a shock or surprise. This is the Kubler-Ross five stage model originally developed to describe bereavement (Kubler-Ross, 1969). Because of my background in systems' change management, I am more familiar with the SARA model which was adopted from Kulber-Ross. Essentially, it's the same set of stages that one must go through when faced with an unplanned and extreme event, and therefore, that's what I shall use to describe the stages of our experience.

SARA stands for Shock, Anger, Resistance and Acceptance. Our behaviour followed the curve perfectly, without us realising it.

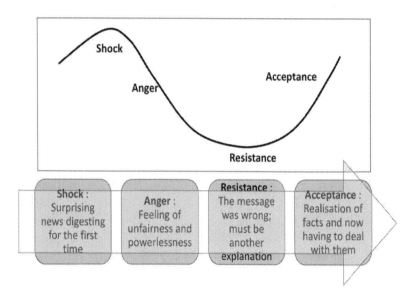

Figure 1 : SARA Curve

In our case:

- Shock – the doctor must be mistaken, too inexperienced, he hasn't considered other options.

- Anger – this stage did not really happen for us as we had decided that the doctor was mistaken and there must be another explanation.
- Resistance – this is where I started looking for other explanations that I could use to disprove the MS assertion.
- Acceptance – due to the resistance, we did not reach acceptance at this time.

A diagnosis of MS is not given (in Scotland) until there are two MRI scans showing lesions. So, at this point we do not have a diagnosis, just a possible cause.

As part of my campaign of resistance I came across a number of articles from chiropractors in Australia that suggested that deformations in the upper spine could give MS like symptoms, particularly blurriness of the eye. It was compelling enough to book an appointment.

The chiropractor took some X rays which clearly showed deformation of the upper spine, probably due to years pouring over computer terminals. My wife undertook a course in spinal correction. Now, I'm not a huge fan of chiropractic therapy due to some of the claims regarding lifestyle enhancement without strong scientific evidence. However, if some benefit could be realised with some skeletal realignment, then I could see little harm.

They say timing is everything. With hindsight this seems to have been the case. In due course the blurriness vanished and the obvious, if wrong conclusion, was that the damage in the upper spine had been causing the problem. This reinforced, again incorrectly, that the young doctor was mistaken in his initial diagnosis.

The eye blurriness was much like having back ache. When it's there you really notice it and it's debilitating. As soon as it's 'fixed' then all memories of discomfort are forgotten, and life returns to normal. Our life went back to normal. Our judgment skewed by the coincidence of the blurriness relapse ending and the course of treatments at the chiropractor concluding. So much so, it never occurred to us to ask for a follow up MRI scan as we were convinced all was well.

Hillwalking

It's little things you notice, again always in hindsight. We used to hill-walk. Not all the time, but a few weekends in the summer. I guess the first things I noticed was a slight increase in cautiousness in my wife when negotiating marshy ground. It's hard to actually describe the change, but all I can characterise it as being 'less fleet of foot' than before.

On one occasion we were coming down a particularly steep slope and she just froze. All she had to do was make a small jump, but clearly something in her brain was inhibiting the movement. Much as I tried to persuade that I would catch her, her defence mechanisms were protecting her from making a movement that perhaps she could not control.

That was the last time we hill walked. This was about three years before formal diagnosis.

Dizziness

About a year before the diagnosis, she started experiencing a sensation of dizziness. This was most pronounced when she went to her gym.

The first visits to the local doctor suggested that there may an inner ear issue. This led to ear syringing, which on the whole was a slightly discomforting experience. Needless to say, this had no impact on the dizziness, but the process of doctors' visits necessarily took some time. This did not stop us from doing anything. Working, going on holiday, all the usual things. The only thing was that on occasion my wife would want my arm for support if the path was steep or uneven. All of this could easily be explained by an inner-ear problem. Therefore, we did not worry too much.

Weakness

All of this came to an abrupt end whilst visiting the Palace of Versailles. It was a very warm day in June and we had been queueing and walking for hours. Towards the end of the day, as we preparing to leave, my wife announced that she needed to lean against a wall as she felt her legs were about to give way! I knew enough about MS that this was a really bad sign. At that point a lot of the previous pieces of evidence that we had accumulated fell sharply into place. The compelling pattern was complete, over-writing our resistance to the initial suspected diagnosis.

There then followed visits to the doctor and the arrangement for a follow-up MRI scan and lumbar puncture. The results were definitive. Lesions in the brain and a high concentration of white blood cells in the spinal fluid.

In general, neurologists are used to giving bad news. After all, by the time the neurologist is involved there are few treatments left. To be fair, our consultant spent a lot of time explaining what could be done with the medications available. We had a few questions, but mainly sat in relative silence while we acquiesced to the final section of the SARA curve, and contemplated that our life, as we knew it, was over.

As I said, hindsight is a wonderful thing. I often wonder what we would have done differently had we recognised the building pattern of evidence. Should we have insisted on a second MRI a year after the first? Clearly, that would have been sensible, but since our life was 'normal' and we were in denial then our behaviour was probably not that unusual. Would an earlier diagnosis have helped? It's difficult to say as MS can remain benign for years. The most constructive view is to say, 'we are where we are' and try to move on. The downside of hindsight is trying to re-live the past, to identify any point where we missed the initial signs of symptoms and perhaps have been able to do something about it. A process that's unproductive, impossible, and therefore, should be avoided.

3. The Treatment

Having received the news in October 2015, the national health service (NHS in the UK) swings into action with their established protocols. This is dependent on the type of MS diagnosed. In our case it was the more common relapsing-remitting multiple sclerosis (RRMS).

The usual course of treatment is to provide disease modifying drugs. In this case immunosuppressant or immune-modification medication. These are designed to suppress or modify parts of the immune response in an attempt to reduce the auto-immune attacks of MS. Over the past few years there has been steady improvement of this type of medication from the injections of interferon beta drugs to the more palatable oral varieties such as fingolimod or dimethyl fumarate.

Fortunately, my wife was prescribed dimethyl fumarate (trade name Tecfidera). I say fortunate, but I shall describe some of the side effects later.

Let's be clear, there is no cure for MS at this time. All these drugs can do is slow the frequency of relapses with a hope that it will reduce the degenerative damage that each relapse causes. Therefore, the course of action given to my wife was to take the medication and try and get on with your life the best you can!

Medical science has made huge strides over the last couple of hundred years. Unfortunately, along with that progress comes the expectation that everything can be fixed or cured. The reality is that this is not the case. However, putting it into perspective, as my grandfather used to say, "it's not what you do get, it's all the things that you could get, but don't". Certainly, these sage words are a useful sanity check, but they should not prevent one from challenging the establishment and looking for alternative approaches. Just to be clear, other approaches are acceptable only provided that their methods are backed with evidence and they follow the principles of scientific development (see chapter 4).

Before I embark on the story of our treatments, I'll outline the Tecfidera journey.

Side Effects and Risks

Tecfidera is an oral drug taken twice a day in pill form. It is an immunomodulator and it will impact the white blood cell count. Therefore, blood tests have to be taken every six months or so.

You start Tecfidera on a low dose for a couple of weeks before increasing to the full dose. My wife handled the low dose with ease. However, once the dose was increased, she did suffer from nausea, skin flushing, and a severely upset stomach. This lasted for about three weeks and is an experience she would like to avoid going through again.

I have heard that many people find the side effects too unbearable and therefore have stopped this particular treatment. In our case that did not happen, and she started the treatment and waited for her next blood test and MRI to see if there had been any impact. In the UK MRI follow-ups happen on an annual basis. Each one provided the 'semi' good news that there had been no change from the previous. Therefore, the treatment should continue unchanged.

I'm going to add a little hindsight here. Although the MRI did not indicate any change, I felt that there has been a gradual impact on mobility. Not enough to suggest a relapse, nor really enough to accurately measure, but more a 'feeling'. I appreciate this is extremely unscientific, and normally I would try and avoid any such conjecture. Nevertheless, during the first two years since formal diagnosis, with hindsight, I felt that there was a gradual impact.

Exploring Alternatives

The role of partner in this journey can be quite emasculating. It's all very well trying to be supportive, but with no influence the role is reduced to asking how one feels. With repetition, this becomes very annoying, as has been pointed out to me on numerous occasions.

In order to remain involved, I chose to improve my knowledge of MS and available treatments. I was completely realistic in the sense that I did not think that I would suddenly discover a miraculous cure that has eluded the scientific and medical community. I just wanted to understand that we were embracing 'good living' practises that may help rather than relying on just one approach.

However, any search inevitably leads to all sorts of 'cures' and numerous self-help books, particularly with regard to diet and numerous clinics advertising 'hope and opportunity'.

For example, there are a number of places advertising stem cell injections and promising what appears to be miraculous improvements. I have a simple view on life, and that is, if there was a straight-forward treatment that showed significant improvement, then all the various health boards would have adopted it.

Nevertheless, I did discuss this with our neurologist. He did warn us that there had been some incidents of fairly fraudulent behaviour. I'm sure that the majority of clinics do operate the treatments with integrity, however, without repeatable evidence of results then it is difficult to consider them seriously.

The only credible stem cell therapy appears to be Haematopoietic Stem Cell Transplantation (HSCT). This involves harvesting stem cells from the bone marrow. Purifying them in the laboratory. Destroying the patients' immune system with chemotherapy and then re-introducing the purified stem cells into the patients to re-boot the immune system. This is a very high-risk treatment and has only been tried for a few hundred patients worldwide. It is possible to obtain this treatment in a few clinics. However, in our case, and at this time the risks are too high in comparison to the current progression of the disease.

Although our consultants were patient and were willing to discuss the options that I have outlined, it was clear that they had a protocol, and following it was the way it had to be. In all fairness, they do have to deal with numerous patients and in general the prognosis from neurologists is not hopeful. So, they have to prescribe what they feel is best whilst working within the parameters set by the governing health board.

The resulting emotions in our part was one of frustration. We were on a production line of therapy and left to get on with our lives and hope for the best. That's how it was, and we dutifully followed the therapy and tried not to think that our lives, if not over, would be severely curtailed.

About six months later we came across an article in a newspaper that changed our approach. It set me off reading as much as I could trying to understand the available treatments and the underlying nature of the problem. However, before I recount that story it's necessary to give you some background on how the science has evolved and the subsequent rise of the pharmaceutical industry and our dependence upon it. How this dependency influences the treatments that we are offered, and sometimes, not always, limits the range of choices available.

4. The Basis of Science

Science and technology under-pins our society. This has not always been the case, but it is the case in our modern world. In this section, I want to discuss the science that we have come to depend upon. I want to explain why we put our trust in science and not, for example, faith healers. In doing so, I also want to highlight some of the conflicts that exist within our society that sometimes divert us from the best therapies.

The Scientific Method

Let's talk a little about science. To be specific, the scientific method. Basically, the concept is very simple, (1) have an idea (a hypothesis), (2) test the said hypothesis in a series of experiments, (3) publish the results so that others can confirm or contradict your results. If the results can be verified, then it seems likely that the hypothesis was sound and therefore can be accepted. If, on the other hand, the results cannot be verified or repeated then the hypothesis must be rejected. This methodology was first put forward by Francis Bacon in 1621, building on the philosophies of the renaissance thinkers, and has successfully stood the test of time.

A couple of observations. The first is that anyone can come up with an idea. You can be the smartest person in the world, but the idea or hypothesis is fundamentally a guess. Until that guess can be verified by experiment and measurement, that's all it is, a guess. A guess is as valueless as any other guess until it is proven. The second point is a little more subtle, and occurred to me when I was an undergraduate, and for which I need to expand the story a little.

Anyone that takes high school physics will know Ohm's law. Basically, it's the relationship between voltage to current flow in a circuit, and it's essential for any electrical or electronic design. This 'law' was developed empirically, that is, by observation and not from fundamental scientific principles.

At the end of the nineteenth century and the beginning of the twentieth, scientists were beginning to understand the composition of materials and therefore, were eager to explain Ohm's law from first principles. Without going into technical detail, the first model to attempt this was proposed by Paul Drude in 1900. This model was based on the classical understanding of physics, that is, free electrons move like billiard balls. Although the model did indeed give an expression that conforms with Ohm's law there were a number of subtleties with electrical and thermal conductivities that did not agree with experimentation. The initial hypothesis, or guess, had not been quite right.

H.A. Lorentz (1905) refined the model with a distribution of electrons' velocities, and this gave the promise of being able to predict the Hall effect (a transverse voltage with respect to current flow in a material due to an applied magnetic field). However, the validating experimental results still did not agree with the theory. So, again, there was something wrong with the hypothesis.

Over the next 15 years additional refinements were made to the hypothesis to explain the discrepancies from reality. However, all these refinements failed to get to the heart of the matter.

This changed with the advent of quantum mechanics during the mid-1920s. Electrons were not considered as being like billiard balls but having properties that were more 'wave like'. This 'root cause' shift in understanding was a game changer. Without delving into the technicalities, and even making some pretty crude assumptions this new model, the Sommerfeld-Drude model, resolved the discrepancies that had been plaguing the previous ideas.

The epiphany that struck me at that formative age, and has remained with me ever since, is that if your initial idea is wrong, then no matter how much 'tweaking' you do, it will in all likelihood not represent reality. Whereas, if your idea is fundamentally on the right lines, then even with some crude assumptions you should be able to derive some insight and understanding of what is going on. As a famous 19th century philosopher said, 'It is better to be roughly right than precisely wrong' (Read, 1898).

The reason for this diatribe is firstly, to outline the scientific method which has been the basis for improving our understanding in science over the last 400 years. Secondly, to remind us that sometimes we need to reset our original 'guess' to something new and not stick dogmatically to traditional ideas. Of course, any new idea must be subjected to the scientific methodology. As I said before, all ideas are guesses until they are proved by experimentation.

Let's hold onto the thought of trying to understand the 'root cause' of a problem. We'll come back to it later. In the mean-time let's discuss the pharmaceutical industry.

The Growth of Pharmaceuticals

The late 19th and early 20th centuries were an explosion of innovation and ideas, not only in physics, but also chemistry, biology, biochemistry, and astronomy. The ideals of rational thought and experimentation as set out in the scientific method kick started the pharmaceutical industry. Prior to this time pharmacies or apothecaries had provided remedies built upon traditional remedies.

In the mid-19th century a number of key players emerged, such as Beecham who started to patent medicine in 1842 and manufacture it in 1859; the Pfizer company founded in 1849; and Bayer founded in 1863. These companies having their roots in the chemical industry employed the same techniques to develop medicines, although the definition of medicine was fairly loose. The search was on for feel good medicines without the destructive side effects of the opioids such as laudanum. In 1895 Bayer marketed diacetylmorphine, an over-the-counter product, under the trade name Heroin. As we all know that was less successful than originally hoped. Although it did take quite a number of years before the product was banned. Bayer did have a major success commercialising aspirin, and during World War One had its aspirin trademark and its US assets seized by the US government. Thus, it was clear that governments were realising the importance and value of the pharmaceutical industry to the evolving world economy.

The next step change in pharmacy was following the discovery of the penicillin mould in 1928 by Alexander Fleming. The understanding of how to manufacture penicillin on an industrial scale, together with the widescale use during the Second World War to combat battlefield infection and pneumonia, created a new era for the industry. Not only did the companies increase investment in research, develop more anti-biotics, but there also developed a tacit trust from the public in the new 'wonder-drugs'.

Remember the operating principle of any company is to make money for its shareholders. We have already seen that assets and patents can be seized as spoils of war in order to gain commercial advantage. Therefore, it's in the interests of the businesses to patent any or all of the fundamental research to protect that commercial advantage. This is completely reasonable for items that have been developed, but what about naturally occurring substances?

The need to maximise profits can lead to rather shameful and unethical behaviour, not only from business but also from government.

Behaviour and Ethics

In 1932 the US public health service wanted to understand the natural history (from inception to resolution) of syphilis. The six-month project, undertaken in cooperation with Tuskegee University in Alabama, enrolled 600 poor African-American field workers, 399 having had contracted syphilis and 201 without the disease. The subjects were given free medical care, meals and free burial insurance for their participation.

When funding was exhausted after the six months, the project continued. The subjects were not informed. By the mid-1940s penicillin was available and was an effective treatment for syphilis, but none of subjects received this treatment. The most shocking part of this whole affair was that the project was finally terminated, but not until 1972! Only following a leak to the press. Fortunately, as a result of this, strict rules for clinical trials were put in place to protect patient interests. Nevertheless, allowing a trial to run for 40 years, exploiting the poorest in society, has undoubtedly got to be one of the lowest points in the history of clinical trials and, in all probability, severely damaged the trust between the public and the health consortia.

What about business ethics? Consider the drug pyrimethamine. This was originally developed by Nobel Laureate Gertrude Elion at Burroughs-Wellcome as a means to combat malaria. The drug has been available since 1953 and has been used wildly to combat malaria and more recently as part of the treatment of HIV/AIDS. By all reasonable measures this was a successful product, and more importantly, affordable.

The trade name for pyrimethamine is 'Daraprim'. Through a series of sale of rights and acquisitions, Daraprim was bought by Turing Pharmaceuticals in August 2015. The CEO, Martin Shkreli, a former hedge fund manager made the news in September 2015 by raising the cost per dose of Daraprim 5,500%. That is, from $13.50/dose to $700/dose. The manufacturing cost (at that time) was about $1/dose.

Martin Shkreli's defended his actions in an interview with Bloomberg Markets: "If there was a company that was selling an Aston Martin at the price of a bicycle, and we buy that company and we ask to charge Toyota prices, I don't think that that should be a crime."

The danger of unethical pricing of a sole supplier generic drug is very real. This example is not the first and certainly will not be the last. It should, however, act as a warning at some of the practices that can and will be employed in order to maximise profit. Because this is pharmaceuticals, the consequences of over pricing are very real. The vulnerable and dependent people cannot afford to buy the drugs.

In this particular case there was both good and bad news. Martin Shkreli went to jail. Not for overpricing, but for securities fraud in a previous role. The downside is that in the US (as of 2019), Daraprim still cost ~$700/dose! You have to judge for yourself whether the company is behaving ethically[1].

Vitamins

An interesting story is that of vitamins. At the beginning of the 20th century, it was felt that food hygiene could be improved by processing food, either by sterilization or grain polishing and milling. However, although the shelf life of grains and cereals was increased, two common diseases for the time, beriberi and pellagra started to increase.

In 1905, William Fletcher discovered that eating unpolished rice seemed to prevent beriberi. There was something in the husk that prevented beriberi. In 1906, Sir Frederick Gowland Hopkins discovered that

---

[1] In February 2020 the FDA approved the first generic version of Daraprim.

certain compounds present in food were important for health and growth. In 1912, Cashmir Funk called these special nutritional compounds 'vitamine'. 'Vita' means life and 'amine' from the thiamine compound that was isolated from rice husks. Hopkins and Funk developed the vitamin hypothesis of deficiency disease. That is, if one does not receive enough vitamins then illness may result.

This first identified vitamin, thiamine, was called vitamin B1. The race was on. The identification of vitamins came, fairly, thick and fast. Vitamin A in 1914, vitamin B in about 1916, vitamin B2 in 1926, vitamin B6 in 1934, and so on.

In 1922 scientists were trying to find ways to prevent rickets (soft, weak and deformed bones in children). They found that a component of cod liver oil would provide an effective defence. They named it 'vitamin D', only due to the fact that vitamins A,B and C had already been identified. The slight mistake was the fact that this one was not a vitamin, but a hormone.

Nobel prize laureate (awarded in 1928), Adolf Windaus, discovered 'vitamins' D_1, D_2 and D_3. D_1 was a mixture of compounds and hence the term is no longer used. Vitamin D_2 is found in plants exposed to sunlight, whilst D_3 is produced in human skin (and animal fur) exposed to sunlight.

The point is that vitamin D drastically reduced the occurrence of rickets. So much so, that during the 1930 and 1940 food was fortified with vitamin D in the US, UK and other industrialised countries, which proved extremely effective at rickets prevention. However, during the 1950s there was a change in public health policies and vitamin D fortification was banned in the UK and a number of other nations. This was due to some cases of hypercalcemia (calcium poisoning) being observed and there was a suspicion that these may be attributed to the food fortification. Definitive linkage was not proven (Pilz, 2018, Jul 17).

The fortification of food stuffs may have been a sledgehammer to crack a nut. Clearly, vitamin D guarded against rickets, but there was an increasing body of information that it benefited other ailments. Also, the perception now existed within the population that supplements were beneficial. A concept not lost on the pharmaceutical industry.

In order to maximise profits by limiting competition it is necessary to own the product. In fact, the process of increasing the vitamin D content of foodstuffs was successfully patented in 1923, leading to significant returns for the industry. It was not invalidated until 1943 by the appeals court stating that it was not an invention, but a discovery. The point being, that in order to make and maintain profits the pharmaceutical industry cannot use vitamin D, which is naturally occurring, but must invent or develop other compounds.

The Rise of Additives

The industrial synthesis of vitamins was developed during the 1930s and 1940s. This, together with the public's perception that vitamins were essential for good health, led to birth of the 'health' additives industry. By the 1950s vitamins A, B1, B2, E and K1 were being manufactured and being produced at a price point that made them readily affordable.

The public's perception was enforced when medical professionals such as Roger Williams (Williams, 1956) proposed that each person had differing nutritional needs. This was later re-enforced by double Nobel prize laureate, Linus Pauling. Pauling advocated that daily doses of vitamin C would reduce the incidence of catching a cold or flu (Pauling, 1976). It should be noted that Pauling's claims have been scientifically tested many times, using double-blind sample populations, and have shown that supplementation with vitamin C does **not** prevent colds (Anderson, 1972, Sep 23 107(6)). Additionally, Pauling claimed that high doses of vitamin C were an effective treatment for certain cancers. Claims also debunked by researchers (Borst, 2008 Dec 2; 105(48)).

Nevertheless, although Pauling claims about vitamins were not accepted by the scientific community, some were largely accepted by the public. The prestige of a scientific heavyweight significantly contributed to the increased consumption of vitamin C and the ongoing, and incorrect, belief that the more one takes then the better one will be protected.

The irony is that most of us do not need any supplement if we have a properly balanced diet. We should be able to ingest most of our needs directly from food, with the possible exception of vitamin D, which requires sunlight. If there is an underlying deficiency, then taking supplements is an acceptable way to boost one's level. Provided it is recommended by a medical professional. Taking too much of the water-soluble vitamins, C and Bs, will only result in expensive urine, as the body will take what it needs and will then secrete the excess. Too much fat-soluble vitamins, A, D, E and K could lead to a vitamin build up in the liver, which is undesirable. Another reason why supplements should be prescribed only if there is a need.

In the US, roughly $30Bn/year is spent on supplements. In the UK, it's a mere £400m/year (both 2016 figures). The global supplement market is expected to grow at 6.9% between 2020 and 2025. With this sort of money to be made, it would be reasonable to expect business to try and exercise control in order to maximise their profits. After all, as we have seen, they need to manufacture compounds to make money (by patenting), rather than package discovered compounds.

It therefore, should come as no surprise that there are cases of strong influence being made. I really want to avoid conspiracy and conflict of interest theories. There are plenty of publications that criticise the pharmaceutical industry (Angell, 2005). However, it is interesting the amount of money that is spend lobbying regulatory agencies and producing copycat drugs. Just to clarify, copycat drugs are high-cost medicines that cost significantly more than those that they mimic or replace, but are no more effective.

This section was really about how vitamin supplements came about and became imbedded in the psyche of the population at large. It is clear that over the past fifty or so years there has been a perception that we need to take additional vitamins. This has been advocated by some scientists and supported by the industry for the reasons I have outlined. Unless you have a measurable deficiency then taking such supplements is a waste of time and money. As I said earlier, the one possible exception may be vitamin D which is dependent upon the amount of sunlight and therefore can be influenced by location. However, one should be careful of the number of publications that abound advocating large doses of vitamin D without medical supervision, with limited, if any, detailed evidence of benefit. This 'quackery' could be misleading as a minimum or dangerous in the extreme.

I shall now recall how a started this chapter, the scientific method. Anyone can have a hypothesis (a guess), but it's repeatable evidence that makes it science. Just because someone says that taking vitamin supplements is a good idea is not evidence that it is actually required. If, however, measured deficiencies are detected and a medical professional recommends supplements, based on the evidence, then that would be a good reason to take them.

Of course, like everything in this evolving story, the medical profession has changed throughout recorded history as our knowledge has improved.

Evolution of the Medical Practitioner

The Greek physicians believed strongly in balancing the four humours (c500 B.C.). That is, blood, yellow bile, black bile and phlegm and good health is achieved when they are in the correct proportions with one another. It is interesting to note that Indian Ayurvedic medicine had developed a concept of three humours even earlier than this.

The Romans were highly influenced by the Greeks and witnessed the establishment of hospitals, the earliest being built in the 1st century A.D. Archaeological artefacts including cupping vessels, scalpels, spatula probes, catheters and forceps, to name but a few, have been recovered. This indicates that fairly sophisticated medical regimes were in place. Good diet and the use of herbs as medicines was practised, although some substances such as sulphur, asphalt and animal excrement, used in purification, were perhaps less beneficial.

The Renaissance was the next major step in the journey. Knowledge filtered from the Islamic world on lessening the impact of disease after injury. As legal and cultural restrictions reduced, the dissection of bodies allowed a much better understanding of anatomy. Gradually techniques such as bloodletting, which was used to balance the humours, was stopped as it was realised it did more harm than good.

As a better understanding of the body prevailed, new chemical preparations also became available. Such as quinine, from the bark of the quina tree, or laudanum from opium. These were used in the treatment of malaria and as a painkiller respectively. The medical expertise and the arsenal of available treatments was improving.

During the 18th and 19th centuries the skills of the medic was somewhat different to those required today. The successful surgeon was not one who was empathetic with the patient, but one who could perform accurately and with speed. This was a necessity due to the lack of any anaesthetic. This was probably true at any time up to the inclusion of chloroform in surgery after the 1850s.

This necessity of speed led to one of the strangest stories that entered popular culture, that of Scots surgeon Robert Liston. Liston practised in London and had been described as "the fastest knife in the West End. He could amputate a leg in 2½ minutes".

In his most famous case, he had to amputate the leg of a patient. This he accomplished in less than two and half minutes. While doing so, he accidentally amputated two fingers of his young assistant and slashed the coat tails of a spectator (spectators stood very close to the action at that time). The patient died afterwards with gangrene. The assistant also died later of gangrene. The spectator dropped dead from fright after his coat tails were slashed, seemingly assuming something more vital had been cut.

This remains the only case in history of an operation having a 300% mortality rate!

Fortunately, with the advent of anaesthetics the need for speed diminished. We also see the medical community start to rely more on manufactured medicines rather than natural remedies. As we have seen earlier, the rise of science and in particular physics, chemistry and biochemistry gave rise to the new industry of pharmaceuticals. The medical practitioner now became much more of a scientist utilising the newly produced remedies based on experimental data rather than unproven traditional approaches.

The upside of this is that more people are treated more successfully. So much so that with the development of vaccines, some diseases were effectively eradicated, like smallpox. The more we learn, the greater the chance of finding cures for very complex or multifactorial diseases such as cancer or autoimmune disorders.

The downside, I suppose, is a blind trust in the pharmaceutical industry. Provided the science is sound then I would not have any issue, but as I have shown, sometimes the behaviour and ethics can be questionable. I am not suggesting for a moment that any medical practitioner would provide a patient with bad guidance, but their options may be limited by what is presented to them by the pharmaceutical industry and health boards.

In summing up this chapter I wanted to highlight that it's important for the reader or patient to be guided by their medical practitioner, but to remain vigilant and always question their reasoning. There is a saying that 'there are no stupid questions'. Therefore, it's perfectly reasonable to challenge the logic of any particular medication or treatment. To be fair, in my experience, the professional practitioner has been more than happy to provide clear and full answers.

5. The Influence of Timing

We're all prisoners of time and timing. Just think of any major event or discovery. It would not have been possible but for the successes and failures of those that went before. That in itself dictates the timeliness of any dependent event. As we saw in the previous chapter, medical science has evolved as the knowledge in anatomy improved and was further enhanced with the development of bioscience and pharmaceuticals. With each development in knowledge or technology the next step was enabled, and an improvement in treatment followed.

Into this progress we now need to factor the story of multiple sclerosis.

First Indications

The first medically documented case of MS was by Jean-Martin Charcot in 1868. He was a French neurologist and was best known for his work on hysteria, which at the time was considered to be a physical illness in females. Fortunately, his ideas about hysteria were later refuted. Nevertheless, based on existing reports and his own observations, he was the first to document a disease that he called 'scierose en plaque', characterised by tremors, slurred speech, abnormal eye movements and post-mortem hardened scar tissue around the nerve fibres. This is generally accepted as being the first documented evidence of multiple sclerosis.

During the latter half of the 19th century more and more evidence of MS was observed, including the fact that it impacted women more often than men, and the symptoms were not consistent. That is, they differed from person to person.

The problem faced by researchers at this time was the availability of tools. Researchers could dissect brain and nerve cells, examine tissue samples under a microscope but had no means of determining where, and more importantly why damage was occurring.

Nevertheless, the researchers persevered, gathering information and trying to make sense of the observational data that was becoming available.

It took until the middle of the 20th century before step changes in knowledge were possible. In 1953 Crick and Watson discovered the structure of DNA. This was the beginning of a whole new branch of science, genetics. This would prove to be a step change in understanding of how genes regulate the immune system, which in turn would lead to a much more in depth understanding of the immune system itself.

It took until the 1970s before imaging tools were developed that could 'look' inside the body. The first of these, the CT scan (computed tomography scan) used X rays to build up a cross sectional view of the body. Although an important tool, X rays by their very nature can only show differences in density of objects within the body. Thus, limiting their usefulness in soft tissue inspection. The more important development was MRI (magnetic resonance imaging). This also produced cross sectional views of the body, but since it does not use X rays and relies on the absorption of radio frequencies by certain atoms, usually hydrogen atoms, this results in images of the soft tissues of the body, such as the brain. This was a major leap forward. It allowed the medical establishment to have an almost real-time view of what was going on in the body, and for the first time in the brain. The first production MRI scanners started to become available in the early 1980s. That's only 40 years ago!

In effect, we're looking at a disease that the medical community has only had tools to understand what might be going on in the body for less than half a century. With this perspective it could be argued that the level of understanding has come quite a long way in a relatively short time.

As we shall see, armed with these tools it was possible to classify the types of multiple sclerosis.

Multiple Sclerosis Types

By 1996 four varieties of MS had been classified. These are Relapsing Remitting MS (RRMS), Primary Progressive MS (PPMS), Secondary Progressive MS (SPMS) and Clinically Isolated Syndrome (CIS).

Clinically Isolated Syndrome

Let's start with Clinically Isolated Syndrome (CIS). This refers to the first event that a patient experiences. Typically, a person experiences a single symptom such as the blurriness in an eye. Sometimes it could be multiple symptoms, such as eye blurriness and tingling in the legs. The episode is usually followed by a complete or partial recovery.

This was exactly the pattern that my wife exhibited. If I had known that a person experiencing CIS who also has a brain lesion has a 60% - 80% chance of an MS diagnosis within several years, then that would have probably modified my behaviour. In all likelihood, we would have remained in denial, but being armed with more information may have helped us to reach the acceptance phase of the SARA curve in a more-timely manner. As I said before, hindsight makes us all experts.

Relapsing Remitting MS

This is by far the most common type of MS with which most patients, including my wife, are initially diagnosed. Approximately 80% of those diagnosed with MS are categorised as having RRMS.

The disease is characterised by the patient having an 'attack' which is then followed by a period of no apparent disease activity (remission). The duration between attacks is completely unpredictable. The remission interval could be months or even years. An attack is characterised by a new symptom. A schematic of the RRMS timeline is shown below.

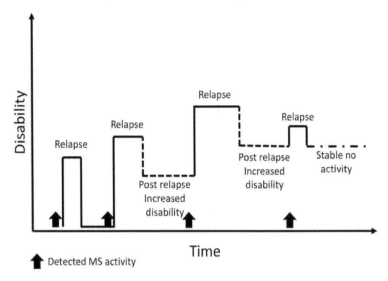

Figure 2 : RRMS Progression

Following a relapse or attack, there may be partial or complete recovery of the symptoms, which can lead to falsely believing that there is no illness. However, with successive relapses it is likely that the disability will increase, with some symptoms becoming permanent.

Primary Progressive Multiple Sclerosis

Primary Progressive MS affects about 10-15% of MS sufferers. It is characterised by increasing disability from the outset. There may also be increasing disability without any detected worsening neurological functions. Hence the progressive name. A schematic of a PPMS time line is shown below.

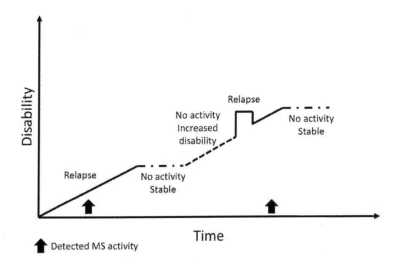

Figure 3 : PPMS Progression

PPMS differs from other types of MS is where the damage occurs. More damage occurs in the spinal cord than in the brain. This makes PPMS more difficult to diagnose and treat.

Secondary Progressive Multiple Sclerosis

RRMS often continues to worsen, but instead of relapse and remission, a steady progression of worsening symptoms takes hold. This is called Secondary Progressive Multiple Sclerosis. A number of people with RRMS eventually transition to secondary progressive MS. Studies indicate that 10% of RRMS sufferers reach SPMS after 5 years, increasing to 25% after 10 years and 75% after 30 years (Tremlett, 2008 Apr 14(3)). A schematic of the progression from RRMS is given below.

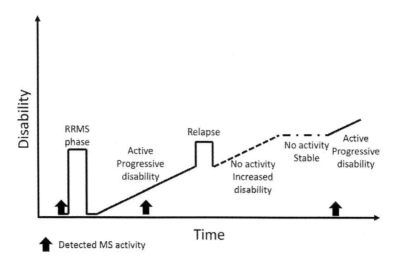

Figure 4 : SPMS Progression

When or why the transition occurs appears to be not understood. The good news, such that it is, is that disease modifying drugs do seem to reduce the number of people making the transition.
Nevertheless, when I read how this progressed, I was extremely disheartened. It seemed that the key task was to try to avoid relapses. If these could be reduced, then the probability of at least remaining within the RRMS phase seemed greater, and therefore, the

chances of moving to the SPMS phase would be reduced.

Optimistic Time?

Maybe I'm being optimistic, but timing is everything. If it had not been for the development of CT and MRI scanners in the 1960 and 1970s, identifying the differences between the variants of multiple sclerosis would not have been possible. It would not be possible to monitor what's going on in the brain and spine, and therefore, to monitor the effects of the myriad of drug treatments that would gradually be developed. All in all, we're in a much better place than we were 50 years ago, although there are still many unknowns.

In addition, the creation of on-line libraries has meant that anyone, suitably motivated, can find information to help their understanding and to aid their decision making.

It was such a trawl that led us to a fairly innocuous article in a newspaper that changed our lives.

6. A New Hope

The article was published in the Daily Mail (Gornall, 2016) and told the story of George Jelinek, a Melbourne neurologist, who had brought his own MS under control. He was given the bad news that he had MS in 1999, and like us, was impacted with the same level of denial, despair and sense of hopelessness that my wife and I had faced.

However, in this case, fate dealt a fortuitous blow. He came across a paper in the Lancet medical journal. The paper was called 'Effect of low saturated fat diet in early and late cases of multiple sclerosis' (R.L. Swank, 1990) and was a long-term study of MS patients over a 34 year period. The conclusion being that those who followed a very low-fat diet showed significantly less deterioration than those who did not.

He says in the article that "when I read it I almost wept". This gave him the evidence to continue the research and look for connections that others had missed, to identify further lifestyle changes and in so doing he became his own guinea pig. This is not an overnight miracle cure. It's a change to lifestyle and therefore takes a lot of time. Particularly since MS has been attacking the immune system probably for a significant period of time before detection. In Jelinek's words, "it took years for the symptoms to disappear …, it was gradual, but seven years after diagnosis I realised I no longer had them".

Just to be clear, George Jelinek holds the position of professor, and is the founder of the Neuroepidemiology Unit in the Melbourne School of Population and Global Health. He is well respected in his field and had published his research in 'Overcoming Multiple Sclerosis' (Jelinek, 2016). The book is extensively researched, and without putting too fine a point on it, once both my wife and I had read it, **it changed our lives**. I would recommend this for all people suffering from MS.

The Jelinek Approach

I am not going to describe Jelinek's book, there's little value that I could add, and I doubt I could convey the message as well as he does. What I'm going to describe is how we approached his methodology, what worked for us and what, we felt, was less successful and why. Then how this spurred me to do additional research that modified my wife's treatment.

There are seven steps to Jelinek's recovery programme, although it's only the first five that actively influence the disease. These are:

- Eat well
- Get plenty of sunshine and vitamin D
- Take regular exercise
- Meditate
- Take prescribed medication if needed

What I am going to do is to consider the above five stages and explore the logic and facts that Jelinek highlighted, and the rationale we employed to apply the lessons in our journey.

Diet

The comprehensive and fundamental work was carried out by Roy Swank who followed 144 MS patients on a low-fat diet for 34 years. The results were published in the Lancet in 1990 (R.L. Swank, 1990). If the original paper doesn't excite you then have a look at the Swank MS Foundation website (http://www.swankmsdiet.org). Roy Swank was a highly respected neurologist with a large number of academic publications and honours.

Quoting from the discussion of the paper, "our findings indicate that a diet of ≤20 g saturated fat daily was best able to keep patients with MS ambulant and working when it was started before the patients' normal abilities and activities were restricted - under these circumstances about 95% of MS patients remained only mildly disabled for approximately 30 years".

Basically, Swank identified a high correlation between saturated fat intake and MS mortality. Put simply, the more saturated fats absorbed by the body the greater the impact on MS disabilities. This sounds really encouraging. All that needs to be done is stick to an ultra-low-fat diet, and hopefully the rate of disease progression will be reduced and therefore becomes manageable. It should be noted that Swank's protocol eliminated saturated animal fats but added unsaturated fats from fish and vegetable oils.

Of course, as I outlined in the chapter about the scientific method, the acceptance on any hypothesis has to be backed up with repeatable experimental evidence. Here we come up against two problems. The first is time duration. Trying to repeat an evidence gathering process that lasts 30 years is somewhat daunting. Unless a number of experiments are carried out in parallel then the earliest that comparable results will be available is in 30 years! The second is people. Trying to persuade a group of individuals to lead a highly restrictive lifestyle when there are other approaches available is a big ask. The other approaches I'm referring to are disease modifying drugs. It's hard, nae impossible, to reproduce the conditions of Swank's work since at that time disease modifying drugs were not available. Trying to persuade a group of volunteers to give up their medication, which they had been told is the best treatment available, in order to be part of a long-term experiment that may or may not yield positive results, is problematic.

An example of this is recent work to reaffirm the role of a low-fat diet on MS, specifically on brain MRI measures (Yada, 2015). The results of the study showed no change in MRI scans in the set of volunteers. One of the reasons of the lack of results was suggested may be due to the patients use of disease modifying drugs and a small sample set of volunteers, 61 in this trial.

The biggest problem with Swank's work was that it was conducted before the days of formally randomised trials, and as such has faced resistance from the medical and scientific establishment. Is this fair? Surely common sense, and the evidence that the vast majority of patients who followed the low-fat diet did have much better health than those who did not, is compelling evidence that fat does influence the MS mechanisms.

So much so, that ongoing large population studies continue that do support Swank's findings. For example, a study of MS mortality by latitude and diet (Esparza M.L., 1995; 142(7)) clearly shows a trend of decreasing mortality as the ratio of unsaturated and saturated fats increases.

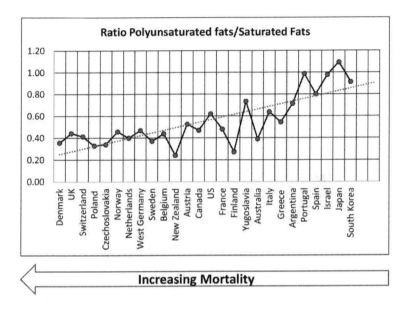

Figure 5 : MS Fat Consumption by Country

Using figures from Esparza et al.

Let's look at one more example. Professor Jelinek has continued to investigate the effects of diet on MS disabilities (Hadgkiss, 2015) on a population of almost 2500 volunteers. The best way to convey the results is to quote from the conclusion section:

"This study supports a strong and significant association between dietary habits and MS outcomes, in particular quality of life and level of disability. A higher intake of fruit and vegetables and healthy fat intake appear to be important dietary factors, while dairy and meat consumption require further investigation."

Again, a compelling argument, albeit not perfect. However, there does seem to be strong evidence that saturated fats have a negative impact on MS. That was enough for us. It seemed sensible to modify our diets. At the very least it could do no harm, cutting fat out of one's diet has obvious health benefits irrespective of having MS.

My wife, and myself in support, embraced the diet. This basically meant we became pescatarians and removed all meat and dairy from our diets. To be honest, I struggled with dairy. However, I reduced my intake to allow myself one cappuccino and one yogurt, once a day. We were surprised to find the array of nut-based alternatives to replace dairy spreads. We settled on cashew nut spread as a replacement for butter. In addition, we both augmented our diet with linseed oil as a means of increasing our polyunsaturated fat intake. The linseed, which is high in omega 3, was easy to take either in soup or drizzled across a salad.

We also found a local group of like-minded MS sufferers that followed Professor Jelinek's diet who meet up fairly regularly to offer support, advice and compare notes.

Sunshine and Vitamin D

The argument for sunshine and by implication vitamin D has been well established. It has been known for some time that MS rates away from the equator are far higher than those on or near zero degrees. In fact, as can be seen in the following graph of MS mortality rates, in general, as one moves further from the equator the mortality rate increases almost linearly. Of course, there are anomalies. Differences in genetics, diet and even altitude can impact lifestyles, and therefore absolute comparisons are not always possible. Nevertheless, there does appear to be a significant trend.

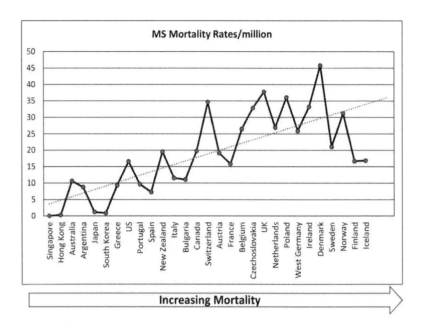

Figure 6 : MS Mortality by Country

Using figures from Esparza et al.

So, it seems likely that sunlight is good for MS sufferers and in particular the vitamin D that is produced from sun exposure. Interestingly, it's been observed that a significant number of MS sufferers appear to have lower than normal vitamin D levels (Mokry, Aug 25, 2015).

As we discussed earlier vitamin D or more specifically vitamin D_3, is not a vitamin but a hormone. It is created by the body as a result of being exposed to sunlight. The actual process is a bit tortuous, which I have tried to show in the following diagram.

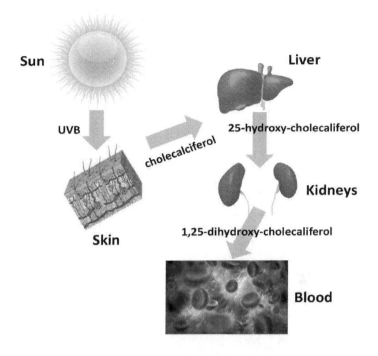

Figure 7 : Vitamin D3 Production

Basically, sunlight strikes the skin. The UVB light energy stimulates a chemical in the skin converting it to cholecalciferol or vitamin D_3. This is then processed by the liver and then the kidneys to finally form 1,25 dihydroxy-cholecalciferol. This is the active form of vitamin D_3.

A couple of things should be noted. Since the process starts with skin absorption, then skin colour is a factor. Dark skin is better at protecting itself against damage. The melanin that causes pigmentation protects the body against UV light and therefore, absorbs less energy than fairer skin. The downside is that darker skin will produce less vitamin D_3 per exposed area of skin. Also, the production of vitamin D is not continuous. Sitting out in the sun for hours on end will not produce more vitamin D than exposing oneself for about 30 minutes or so (assuming strong sunlight). However, exposing more skin area will increase the amount of vitamin D produced. The ideal scenario would be to sunbathe exposing as much of the body as modesty allows each day for about 30 minutes in strong sunlight (more time if the sunlight is less strong).

Unfortunately, as shown in the graph above, MS is more prevalent in countries farther from the areas where there is no strong sunlight. This is clearly evident when one lives, as my wife and I do, in Scotland.

In fact, even within the UK there is clear distribution in MS cases as one moves north, from about 3 per 100000 in England to 10.5 per 100000 in Orkney (Swingler, 1986;49). That's a three-fold increase! Remember, these are the facts, and although all facts are open to interpretation, they do suggest a striking story. The reasons for the increase in prevalence may be many-fold, but surely, given what we already know about MS distribution the argument that it is impacted by sunlight seems compelling.

This was really the 'light-bulb' moment for me. Professor Jelinek advocates taking vitamin D supplements as a preventative measure in his book and goes into a lot more detail on how vitamin D could not only be preventative but may slow progression. The key question is how much vitamin D should one take?

For years the maximum recommended dose of vitamin D_3 was no more than 400iu (international units) per day due to the perceived risk of toxicity. As I mentioned, in chapter 4, when I talked about the initial discovery of vitamin D_3 and the budgets involved in the additive industry. One could speculate that there may have been vested interests, that lobbied to keeping the recommended level of vitamin D_3 intake low in order to promote alternatives.

Professor Jelinek suggests that 10000iu/day would be perfectly reasonable with minimal risk. Fortunately, over the years there have been many studies into how vitamin D_3 impacts MS. It appears that the guidance of 400iu is far too cautious. Patients can absorb much higher doses (Kimball, 2007 Sep;86(3)) without experiencing any ill effects. The study increased vitamin D_3 dosage from 4000iu/day to 40000iu/day in 12 patients during a 28 week period, without exhibiting signs of hypercalcemia (vitamin D poisoning).

The second key piece of data that caught my eye was a study involving 156 patients with RRMS (Pierot-Deseilligny, 2012 5(4)). Basically, the research showed that for every 10 nmol/L increase in vitamin D_3 within the body there was a reduction in relapse rate of 13.7%.

This was interesting. If this was true, then surely all one had to do was increase the amount of vitamin D_3, within safe limits, and relapses could be eliminated. Unfortunately, it wasn't to be a simple as that, as the research did suggest that there was a law of diminishing returns. The relapse rate was reduced but tended to plateau at high levels of vitamin D_3. Nevertheless, this was something that needed pursuing, which I did, and we shall discuss in a later chapter.

Regular Exercise

I have lost count of the number of times that doctors' solutions to almost any ailment is to 'take plenty of exercise and eat fresh fruit and vegetables' (I'm paraphrasing). On the other hand, as our lifestyle has become more sedentary it is clear that we do not tend to keep our bodies in optimal condition. This is particularly apparent in western societies with the rise in obesity and associated chronic illnesses like diabetes, heart disease, strokes and various types of cancers.

In the case of multiple sclerosis, the wisdom used to be to avoid anything that may risk injury and aggravate their symptoms. Therefore, exercise tended to be very limited in nature. The trouble with that approach was that without exercise the body does lose strength and there is a decrease in overall energy levels.

Fortunately, that approach has been discredited and numerous studies from as far back as 1974 by Professor Ritchie Russell (Russell, 1976) to the present day (Halabchi, 2017; 17:185) indicate that exercise is beneficial, particularly aerobic and resistive regimes.

More recent research (Malkiewicz, 2019; 16:15) suggests that physical exercise may improve the stability of the blood brain barrier (which we shall discuss in the immune system chapter), which has got to be good thing, but the caveat is that their research study group was not of sufficient enough scale that definitive conclusions could be drawn.

Of course, there are conflicting studies, such as one about aerobic exercise not improving memory function (Baquet, 2018;6:e6037). The study group was of 77 patients, but the duration of the trial was only 12 weeks. The results indicated no overall conclusion.

My own view is to be suspicious of trials that have small sample groups or short durations. The one thing we do know about MS is that, in general, it is a slow progressing disease. Also, we have seen from Swank and later from Jelinek that sample groups should be large and trials should last a significant time.

There is a lot of information out there which I'm not going to repeat, but we realised that if we were going to address this illness then regular exercise needed to be factored into the equation. Anyway, even common sense suggests that some exercise is not a bad thing and actually promotes a feeling of well-being. At the very least, it's important not to vegetate and not to feel the disease is winning. It's a question of taking control.

To be fair, we did modify the gym routine. One of my wife's on-going symptoms was one of balance. She often joked that 'she walked like a drunk'. Therefore, the treadmill was replaced with the cross-trainer to ensure that the risk of a fall was reduced. My wife continued with weights and rowing to keep her strength up, and in general, putting me to shame for not showing the same dedication. Swimming was a good alternative, providing strengthening as well as aerobic exercise with little or no risk of damage.

An additional exercise regime we adopted was yoga. I shall discuss more of this later, but from rather shaky beginnings we improved to the point that my wife was able to perform the balancing exercises and head stands. I have no evidence on the specific benefits of yoga, but the ability to hold balance was a major boost to her confidence. For my part, I partook in the yoga and we were able to encourage and correct each other to attain the correct poses.

So, with a few adjustments, regular exercise was maintained. Ideally this should have been conducted in the sunshine, but as I have stated already, living in the northern hemisphere has its challenges.

Meditation

Everyone involved with MS says that stress is bad and should be avoided as a possible trigger for a relapse. Why should that be, let's examine the logic and the evidence?

Stress is an integral part of the body's evolved fear response. That is, when placed in a danger situation, whether to fight or run (flight). The body doesn't know what the decision will be so has to prepare itself. The most effective defence is to prepare for the worst and hope for the best. That's what the body does.

Adrenaline is released, the heart rate increases, blood pressure rises, and blood vessels dilate in readiness to supply increased amounts of blood to muscles. At the same time additional chemical messages are released to prime the immune system in readiness for possible injury. It's a very sophisticated process and one that has served us well as we evolved. However, a response that has taken eons to evolve cannot change to deal with the fairly 'safe' lifestyle that has persisted for the last few centuries.

So, we have a situation where in everyday life stress can trigger elements of the body's fear response. The key question is – can this response impact MS? There is substantial evidence that suggests that stress can directly precipitate or worsen symptoms by activating autoimmune cells (Karagkouni, 2013, Aug;12(10)).

Fortunately, there has been quite a lot of work looking into different non-intrusive therapies that can alleviate stress. Also, fortunately, there have been a number of reviews that have sought to examine the broad body of evidence and to summarise their findings. One such piece of work is by Angela Senders and colleagues (Senders, 2012; 2012:567324) that brings together studies in mediation, yoga, hypnosis, biofeedback, Tai chi, relaxation techniques and mindfulness.

As the authors pointed out, not all the studies reviewed were of high quality, usually due to small numbers of patients involved or the assessments could not be shown to be without bias. Nevertheless, without repeating the conclusions verbatim, a number of useful points can be made from the ten (10 out of initial 106 screened for review) higher-quality studies reviewed.

Therapy	Helpful for MS symptoms
Mindfulness based stress reduction	Depression, anxiety, fatigue, quality of life
Relaxation	Quality of life
Yoga	Fatigue
Biofeedback	Bladder incontinence

I had difficulty with the 'quality of life' description as this encompasses so much and is not a clear measure. Fatigue, anxiety, mobility and incontinence are all factors in quality of life. However, from our own experience, yoga was indeed beneficial. Mainly by improving balance. Since my wife was also attending a gym two to three times a week it was not possible to judge whether the yoga helped with her fatigue.

Our own local health service in the UK promotes mindfulness to help with MS. She did attend a number of sessions and practices meditation when at home. She also encouraged me to do it. I had difficulty in clearing my mind and stopping it from wandering. Perhaps if I had focused on it more, then I too would have reached that point of inner calm, but it was something that eluded me. Either that or I wasn't sufficiently motivated.

All in all, it seems that mindfulness or meditation provides some benefits, probably more preventative by keeping stress levels as low as possible. It has also become sufficiently mainstream that health authorities are advocating this type of therapy. Yoga like any exercise, as discussed in the previous section, is probably beneficial. The good thing is there are many types of yoga from highly energetic ones to those that concentrate on more gentle postures and breathing exercises. The important thing is to find one that is suitable to your capabilities and needs. The biofeedback is particularly specialised and concerned with training the pelvic muscles. Fortunately, this was not required, but it's good to know that there are potential treatments if required.

Keep Taking Prescribed Medication

Professor Jelinek describes at length the various types of treatments available to MS sufferers.

There are three basic types of treatment available. These are disease modifying drugs (DMDs) and have the effect of modifying the behaviour of the immune system. The first type is the beta interferons and are immunosuppressants. These have been prescribed for RRMS for 20 years or so (depending on the approving authority) and are injected by the patient. Like most drugs, there are side effects that range from mild flu like symptoms to diarrhoea and vomiting. They work by suppressing the immune response. That is, reducing the number of white cells produced and therefore, reducing the number of cells available to cross the blood brain barrier into the central nervous system to cause damage.

Beta Interferon	Method	Frequency	Side Effects	Expected Benefit
Avonex	Inject into muscle	Once a week	flu like symptoms injection site reaction headache diarrhoea, nausea and vomiting difficulty sleeping hair loss depression decrease in white cells	Reduce the number of relapses by ~30% Little evidence that it slows rate of disability (Shirani & al., 2012;308(3))
Betaferon	Inject under skin	Every other day		
Extavia	Inject under skin	Every other day		
Plegridy	Inject under skin	Once a fortnight		
Rebif	Inject under skin	Three times a week		

The second type are classified as immunomodulators. The difference being that they don't suppress the immune system, but modify the level of response in a number of areas. These are more recent additions to the MS arsenal. The earlier drugs were injection, but the more recent ones can be taken orally. Like the suppressant DMDs they also exhibit side effects but their impact on the disease is supposed to be better. See the table below.

Immuno-modulator	Method	Frequency	Side Effects	Expected Benefit
Copaxone	Inject under skin	Daily or three times per week	injection site reaction	Reduce the number of relapses by ~30%
Brabio	Inject under skin		headache nausea, chest pain, depression, anxiety, gastrointestinal changes	
Aubagio	Oral	Once a day	Feeling sick, diarrhoea, hair thinning, decrease in white cells, skin rash	Reduce the number of relapses by ~50%
Tecfidera	Oral	Twice a day		
Gilenya	Oral	Once a day		
Mavenclad	Oral	Treatment course		

The third type of DMD are aimed at those patients with highly active MS symptoms as the side effects tend to be more serious and can lead to complications and secondary autoimmune problems. There also appear to be higher risks of relapse if the treatments are stopped.

Immuno-modulator	Method	Frequency	Side Effects	Expected Benefit
Mavenclad	Intravenous infusion	Two treatment courses 12 months apart	Infusion-related reactions, increased risk of infection, thyroid problems, skin rash, dizziness, shivering, herpes infection	Reduce the number of relapses by ~70%
Ocrevus	Intravenous infusion	Once every six months		
Tysabri	Intravenous infusion	Monthly in a clinic		
Lemtrada	Intravenous infusion	Two treatment courses 12 months apart		

As we are often told, there is no cure for MS. All of the above attempt to interrupt and slow down the progression. Some claim to improve the level of disability, but there is scant evidence of this.

Our Adoption of Jelinek's Methodology

After diagnosis, my wife was prescribed Tecfidera which is supposed to reduce the chances of a relapse by about 60% and is felt to be one of the best DMDs available for RRMS. As I mentioned already, the downside is that the initial side effects are unpleasant. A number of patients cannot manage the side effects, gastro-intestinal discomfort, diarrhoea, nausea and vomiting. Fortunately, for my wife, these passed after about a month. However, putting this in perspective all we are talking about is a reduction in chance. So, 60% of MS sufferers are likely to see a reduction in MS relapses, but 40% will not see any benefit!

Don't get me wrong, I'm not suggesting that the drugs should be avoided, but pointing out the reality that a reduction in chance is not a guarantee that relapses will reduce.

Also, when I looked into the mechanism of how Tecfidera worked, I could not find any definitive statement. All I could find was that 'the way Tecfidera works is not fully understood …', and that 'it **may** work in two ways: reducing the inflammation when the immune system attacks myelin[2]; and protects nerve cells from damage caused by chemicals released during the immune attack'.

Not exactly a ringing endorsement.

As discussed earlier, the first key point is to reduce (or ideally cut out) saturated fat. We had not been huge meat eaters, so it was relatively easy to remove meat (red meat and chicken) from our diet and stick to vegetables and fish. In addition, my wife removed all dairy from her diet, firstly because of the fat content,

---

[2] the fatty coating that surrounds the 'wires' (axons) in the nervous system

but also secondly, due to the high correlation between milk consumption and MS (Malosse, 1992; 11(4-6)). Trying to understand the mechanisms involved is quite complex, however, it appears that proteins in milk are sufficiently similar to part of the myelin structure and therefore, could potentially trigger an immune response. However, the evidence is limited (von Geldern, 2012 : 8), and clearly many other factors are involved, since a lot more people drink milk than have MS.

Nevertheless, even with little evidence and purely as a risk mitigation strategy, it seemed sensible to remove dairy from the diet. I'll discuss this in a little more detail in the next chapter.

The next change we made was to start taking vitamin D. As soon as we completed reading the book my wife started on 10000 iu/day of vitamin D_3 soft-gels. In fact, I also started taking the supplement, albeit a lower dose. It seemed a sensible defence against the lack of sunlight in Scotland.

Interestingly, the vitamin D story doesn't stop here. This was the beginning of the next stage of the journey that I shall shortly expand upon.

Exercise and mediation were built into our weekly regime. The exercise was fairly straight-forward. Unfortunately, not living in a guaranteed sunny climate, this involved either going to a gym or an indoor swimming pool. The meditation, as I described previously, does suggest some benefits, but frankly, this was one area where I struggled to give support. My wife persevered, but over time that waned as we both became more interested in yoga.

As Jelinek recommended, she adhered to the prescribed medication which we would be following under the guidance of the health service and our local doctor.

Having read as much as I could about Professor Jelinek's approach. Then reading about the role of vitamin D_3 in reducing relapse rates as the concentration in the blood increases. The obvious question is reached. How much vitamin D_3 is required to completely arrest relapses?

However, at this point it is necessary to build a picture of what's happening in the immune system. In reality, I was trying to understand some of the basics whilst we adopted the Jelinek approach. However, to benefit the story, I have decided to insert my understanding at this point in the belief that it will help the subsequent sections fit more logically together.

7. The Immune System

In this section I shall give an overview of the key components of the immune system. This helped me to try to understand the mechanisms that are at work and how potential therapies might modify them. I'm going to try to avoid any complicated medical names as I don't feel they are necessary to conveying the story and can be off-putting to the reader in many cases. However, be aware that the system is extremely complicated, and many scientists spend their entire life trying to understand it. Therefore, it is not possible to explain the detailed functionality in a few short pages, but a glimpse at the salient points. In trying to tell the story, I have tried to refer to published evidence wherever possible. I have also tried to avoid research that has been predominantly focused on the trialling of medications as I felt that such evidence may potentially bias the overall picture. Nevertheless, I have tried to capture the important points that helped me. Hopefully it will help you, the reader, also.

If something in life goes wrong it needs to be corrected. Everything has a tendency to drift from what is considered an optimal condition. Engineers manage this by the use of control systems. That is, if a deviation from the expected condition occurs, then a message or signal is sent to correct the error. This is basic control theory. The body is no different albeit many orders of magnitude more complicated.

If something that should not be there is detected, the body jumps into action sending messages to objects that are designed to handle the invader. Once the invader is dealt with, then the control system can return to the benign monitoring state. At least that's how it should work. However, sometimes things go wrong and to understand that we need to delve a bit deeper into the various mechanisms in the immune system.

The system itself is fantastic. Look at the number of 'nasties' that it deals with on a daily basis, from the moment of the beginning of one's life, right up to one's demise. The immune system has evolved during millions of years to provide the protection that we need to live in a world of pathogens (foreign bodies that causes disease). That's not to say it's perfect. It can occasionally get caught out as media reports of epidemics and pandemics abound, or as diseases evolve or migrate across the species boundary, as with Asian bird flu, AIDS or Covid-19. Nevertheless, it is still extremely effective at dealing with the majority of threats.

The Innate Immune System

The immune system has two key components, the **Innate Immune system** and the **Adaptive Immune system**. The Innate system is found in all plants and animals, although it is more developed in the vertebrates. It provides physical and chemical barriers to infectious agents and has two major components.

The first is called **General factors** and is the first set of defences the body has against an invading foreign pathogen. This can be a physical barrier such as the skin, which is a good tight barrier. Also, the body can secrete enzymes from sweat glands and mucous membranes that provides a barrier to invaders. In addition, the body may exhibit inflammation or a fever response. This is as a mechanism to inhibit the reproduction of viruses or bacteria by making the host environment a more uncomfortable place.

Inflammation releases chemical signals that call up the next level of response, the cellular factors. Everyone will have experienced this basic protection from childhood, generally unaware of the complex processes that underpin it.

Cellular factors, as the name suggests, is really how the body responds to an infection at a cellular level. That is, how it kills a pathogen that has made it through the general factors' first line of defence. Simply put, these are the white blood cells. Specialist types of cells roam around the body, and if they detect a pathogen such as a virus or bacterium, then they kill it. This can be achieved by ingesting the virus or bacterium or releasing chemicals that cause the pathogen to self-destruct. Once a pathogen is detected, chemical messages are released which call up additional white cells to support the fight, which may, in turn, trigger an inflammation or fever response also. These additional chemical messages are important which we shall consider further in the following section.

Even with this very simple introduction, we can see that the immune system is already pretty sophisticated and has a layered defence mechanism. However, the key thing is that the Innate System does not possess an ability to learn. It does not have a memory so that it can be prepared should the same foreign invader attack in the future. This is where the Adaptive Immune system comes in. It is an understanding of this more sophisticated mechanism that is required to appreciate the factors that are at play in multiple sclerosis.

The Adaptive Immune System

The Adaptive Immune system is found mainly in jawed vertebrates. The term adaptive is really the ability to 'remember' a pathogen and hence have the body prepared for any future attacks. As we have already seen the Innate system is complex, and unfortunately this one is also complicated. I shall endeavour to get the salient points across that are necessary for the rest of the story.

The adaptive immune system deals with pathogens in the body's fluids as well as those that have invaded the cells (e.g. viruses). In addition, antibodies are produced and a memory of past infection that allows the immune system to respond very quickly if it is attacked by the same pathogen.

The **Humoral** immune response deals with pathogens in the body, but not in the cells and the **Cellular** immune response deals with pathogens that have invaded the cell structures.

The goal of the humoral response is to produces antibodies. The key thing to note here is that special white blood cells, called B cells, are matured in bone marrow ('B' for bone) and then activated in other organs such as the spleen or lymph nodes. Without going into detail, the B cells produce plasma cells that release antibodies that fight an invading infection. In addition, they also produce B memory cells, so that there is a quicker response to a future attack (of the same pathogen). This process cannot happen without help of additional cells called 'T' cells (after the Thymus where they mature). By binding to the B cells, it is these T cells that help the B cell to proliferate (called differentiation) and mature into antibody producing plasma cells and memory cells. These T cells are imaginatively called T helper cells.

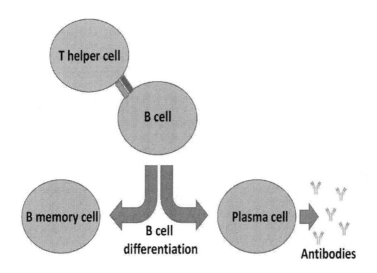

Figure 8 : B Cell Differentiation

Just to recap, the two special white blood cells in the Adaptive immune system are the B cells and the T cells. As we have seen the B cells are required for defence, their primary function, and with the help of T cells, is to replicate (differentiate), thus producing antibodies. These antibodies bind to the invading pathogen, and in turn, attract the specialised white blood cells that can ingest or kill the foreign invader. In addition, they create memory B cells that linger in the body so that any future attack can be quickly recognised allowing the immune system to respond accordingly.

This all sounds good. So, what else do the T cells do?

This is where it becomes interesting. When certain types of white type, including B cells, come across a pathogen they can present a fragment of the foreign body protein on its surface as a signal, called an antigen. For the sake of simplicity, I shall restrict the discussion to B cells.

Think of this antigen as a type of plug like an HDMI plug. Only HDMI sockets can 'fit' it. A USB socket would be useless and therefore ignored. So, in the case of the cell, only a protein that matches the displayed protein fragment can bind to it.

There are a huge number of T cells floating around the body, billions in fact. Each with different antigen receptors (socket). A T cell will only respond when the correct antigen fits the receptor and hence triggers the cell into action.

A T cell that has a receptor that matches the fragment can then bind to the B cell. As I described in the previous section, this is the trigger for the B cell to multiply into plasma cells and produce antibodies. The antibodies flood into the bloodstream and lock onto matching antigens initiating their destruction. Some of the B cells don't produce antibodies but become the B memory cells mentioned earlier.

Clearly, once the 'nasty' has been killed off there is no need for all these antibodies swimming around the bloodstream. Part of the innate system is called the complement system, and one of its roles is immune clearance, that is, clearing up the redundant debris that is no longer required. I add this for background. It's not essential to this part of the story. What is important is to realise that T cells, of a specific kind, can direct and help B cells to destroy the invader.

T Cell Types

There are myriads of what's known as naïve T cells floating around our bodies. When they receive a specific set of chemical messages these naïve T cells are changed into T cells with a specific purpose. There are four main types of T cell. These are **Helper** cells, **Killer** cells, **Memory** cells and **Regulatory** cells. Killer cells form from one specific type of naïve T cell called CD8+, and the others form from a naïve T cell called CD4+. The CD refer to different glycoprotein receptors on the cell surface. This is just a point of interest regarding differentiation and not essential for this story. However, it is important if you wish to research further.

The killer and memory cells are key parts of the active immune system in that they kill off cells that have been compromised by viruses or tumours, and then provide the memory mechanism to guard against future attacks. T memory cells provide a similar function to B memory cells, but are aimed at pathogens that attack cells.

The killer cell is the one that does the work. Basically when, what is known as an immature T cell, encounters an antigen that matches its receptor, it morphs into a killer T cell that is designed to attack cells that have been compromised by the invading antigen. It's more complicated, but for the story that's roughly what happens. It's a killer cell because when it encounters the invader, for example a cell that has been infected with a virus. It attaches to the cell and releases its chemical payload. These chemicals are designed to damage the cell wall (perforin) and kill the virus within (cytotoxins). However, the killer T cell does not work alone and receives instructions from helper T cells. The T helper cells act as co-ordinators. It is these helper cells that drive the adaptive response, and a basic understanding of their actions is needed to complete the immune response picture.

There are numerous different types of T helper cells, but we are going to look at three specific ones and the T regulator cell, and how they are brought into existence.

Creation of T Helper and Regulator Cells

Starting from a naïve T cell, in this case a CD4+ type. Helper cells are created when specific chemical messages are detected. This process is pretty complicated, but essentially any cell that has some sort of foreign material, be it bacteria, virus or a protein that encounters a roaming white cell triggers a response. As mentioned in 'cellular factors', depending on the type of white cell that encounters an invader, chemical messages are emitted.

It had been my intention not to include any complicated chemical names, but actually the picture is clearer if I name some of them. The chemical messages designated 'IL' are interleukin molecules of differing types. 'TGF' is transforming growth hormone, and 'IFN' is interferon.

These stimulate a change in a naïve T cell to be a helper T cell. The type of helper is dependent upon what chemical signals are present. For example, the T_h1 helper cells are designed to fight inter cellular infections such as bacteria, viruses and cancers. So, when a roaming white cell detects a suitable pathogen and, for example, recognises it as a bacterium, in addition to attacking it, it will send out chemical messages to 'ask' for help. If it released IL-12 and IFNα, then T_h1 helper cells would be created.

T_h2 cells are designed to fight parasites. T_h17 cells are designed to combat fungi and extra cellular bacteria (that is bacteria that don't invade cells). A similar process involving different chemical messages would bring these helper cells into the fight.

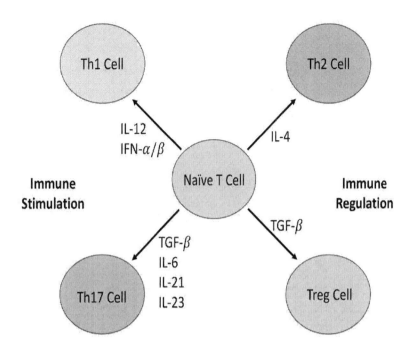

Figure 9 : T Cell Activation (1)

Notice that in some cases it requires a combination of chemical messages to activate a specific T cell (Pennock, 2013 Dec; 37(4)).

Once the helper cells are activated, they do not remain benign. They send out their own set of chemical cocktails to stimulate other cells and thus develop the immune response.

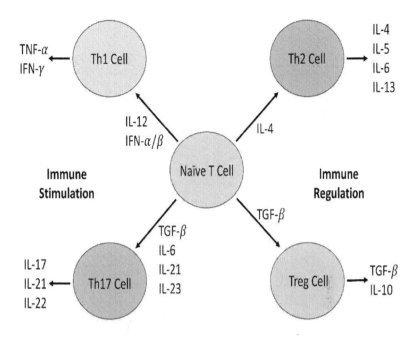

Figure 10 : T Cell Activation (2)

Of course, this is not the whole story. The chemical messages drive further behaviour, but before we look at that, consider the interleukin 4 message (IL-4). IL-4 changes naïve T cells into T_h2 helper cells, which in turn emit IL-4, which will activate more T_h2 cells. This is a positive feedback loop, a self-reinforcing loop. Clearly this mechanism would lead to uncontrollable numbers of T_h2 cells, therefore, a mechanism of control is required to suppress such runaway activation. Fortunately, evolution being what it is, we have such a mechanism.

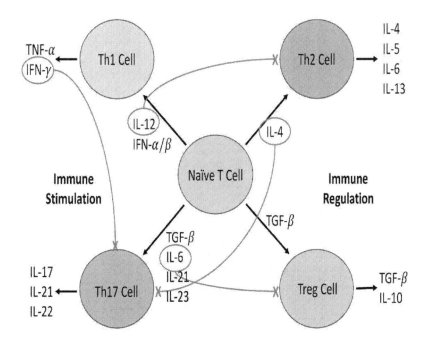

Figure 11 : T Cell Activation (3)

For example, in order to change a naïve T cell into a T_h17 cell all three interleukins shown above, and the transforming growth hormone must be present. However, if IL-4 or IFN-γ is present then the change cannot happen. Similarly, the development of T_h1 helper cells will block the creation of T_h2 cells. Each of the chemical messages ringed blocks the activation of a naïve T cell into one of the helper or regulatory cells. This is the mechanism to ensure this part of the active immune system stays in balance.

T_{reg} (regulator) cells are specifically designed to suppress T cell response and hence limit the immune response. Basically, this provides an overall monitoring and control process. After creating quantities of T cells that stimulate the immune system, it is necessary to close the response down. It would be dangerous for the body to be, for example, constantly running a fever as part of the response. T_{reg} cells are there to prevent the immune system going out of control. In effect to prevent autoimmunity. The number of T_{reg} cells is controlled to be in the 'goldilocks' zone. Not too many, not too few, but just right.

There we have it. A sophisticated control system that identifies foreign invaders, reacts quickly, eliminates the threat and then closes down the response to a benign state in readiness for the next attack. The trouble is, as everyone knows, the more complex the system the more things can and do go wrong. All autoimmune diseases are a symptom of an unwanted immune response. Crohn's disease, psoriasis, rheumatoid arthritis, asthma, type 1 diabetes and multiple sclerosis are all auto immune diseases.

T and B Cells and MS

The brain and central nervous system are supposed to be protected by the blood brain barrier. A semi-permeable layer of cells that protects the brain and central nervous system from pathogens that have entered the body. Obviously in MS this mechanism is not working since it is the myelin within the central nervous system that is being attacked and damaged by the immune system.

The key question is 'what is doing the attacking'. Although an obvious question, it is in fact quite hard to answer. It is first necessary to determine that the patient has MS. Since there is no definitive test for MS it is necessary to use circumstantial evidence derived from spinal fluid (Deisenhammer, 2019, Apr 12) as well as MRI data. Basically, an increased level of antibodies and plasma cells are one of the key indicators that a patient has MS.

The increase in antibodies would naturally suggest that they are responsible for the damage to the myelin. Although there have been no myelin specific antibodies identified, it is suggested that B cells and antibodies may contribute to the development of MS (Weber, 2011, February, Volume 1812, Issue 2). If it's a contribution, then what other mechanisms are at play. As we have seen already, T helper cells are required to allow B cells to proliferate.

It used to be thought that an over-abundance of T_h1 cells was the key driver for MS. In fact, one of the measures to establish MS is the concentration of T_h1 cells found in spinal fluid. Typically, a measure of seven times the normal concentration of T_h1 cells would be one indicator of MS.

In addition to the T_h1 cells, it was felt that T_h2 played a part in the recovery of MS and therefore, it was necessary to ensure balance between these helper cells to control the disease (Nagelkerken, January 1998). However, the picture may be much more complicated. There may be co-operation between flavours of T cell. Damsker, J. et al. (Damsker, 2010, January:1183) reviewed the evidence that suggested that T_h17 cells could be key at driving an immune response as well as, conversely, helping to mediate the T_h1 response.

Other studies have shown that the T_h17 and T_{reg} cells may have a central role in autoimmune activation (Fletcher, 2010, October). As they stated in the paper, **"Indeed, in MS, relapse and remission have been correlated with relative decreases and increases in the frequency of T_{reg} cells"**. In addition, other research seems to indicate a relationship between T_h17 and T_{reg} cells (Nistala, 2009, Volume 48, Issue 6) and increasing

T_h17 cells at the expense of T_{reg} cells trigger autoimmunity (at least in animal models). The mechanisms are complex, but could the imbalance between these types of T cells be the trigger?

More recently, this seems to be borne out by Lee (Lee, 2018, Mar; 19(3)) who states, "many autoimmune diseases are driven by T_h17 cells and suppressed by T_{reg} cells, the balance between these cell types is critically important for pathogenesis, prognosis, and therapy". This is interesting. There does seem to be a picture building for balancing these T cells. It may counter the susceptibility of acquiring an autoimmune disorder and the ability to resist it. Think of it as a set of scales.

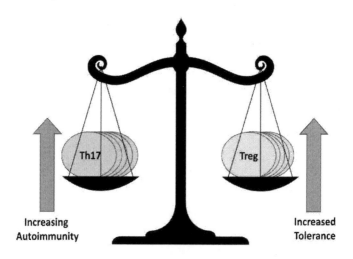

Figure 12 : Th17 and T Reg Balance

An imbalance in favour of T_h17 could promote an autoimmune response. This could be redressed by increasing the T_{reg} cells or suppressing the T_h17 cells. The question is how to achieve the balance?

The obvious answer is to use drugs. One of the mechanisms of beta interferons is to reduce the production of T_h17 cells. More recently the adoption of immune modulators, which work by blocking the immune system signalling, have also been shown to reduce the number of available T cells. Interestingly, one particular drug, Copaxone, is believed to work by flooding the body with proteins that are similar in structure to myelin. The idea being that the drug acts as a decoy and draws the immune response away from the brain and spinal cord.

Recalling that we saw that vitamin D reduces MS relapse rates. What mechanisms are at play, and why should that work? The key ingredient is vitamin D_3 and has been suggested for some time reduce the relapse rate in MS (Munger, 2006 Dec 20;296(23)). As we discussed earlier, this is not a vitamin, but a hormone. That is, a chemical structure that can change the behaviour of cells with which it interacts. There is a wealth of data that supports the facts that vitamin D_3 suppresses the T_h17 cells (Hewison, 2010, June:39(2)), (Chang, 2010, December 10), (Dankers, 2019; 10:1504), (Cantorna, 2015 Apr 7(4)), to name but a few. Of course, suppression is one factor, but what about balance between the T cells? Does vitamin D_3 help balance the $T_h17:T_{reg}$ ratio?

Research around the world is not confined to MS. There is significant work in other autoimmune areas such as type 1 diabetes, rheumatoid-arthritis or lupus. Indeed, some of the papers referenced are from such studies. Provided the underlying mechanisms are the same, even if the diseases that trigger them are different, I believe there is merit in examining their findings.

For example, in women with recurrent pregnancy loss, the ratio of $T_{reg}:T_h17$ and the level of vitamin D_3 was observed to be low (Jinlu Ji, 2019, 23 Mar) and was brought into balance with vitamin supplementation. Similarly, in rodent studies which are often used as a model of human physiology, (Zhang, 2014, Sept., Vol. 8, No. 5) vitamin D_3 is shown to regulate the $T_h17:T_{reg}$ balance.

There is quite a body of evidence that suggests an over-abundance of T_h17 cells drives autoimmunity and that providing vitamin D_3 supplementation helps regulate the imbalance. Would this explain why increased levels of vitamin D_3 reduced MS relapse rates that I mentioned in the previous chapter?

If there was an increase in T_h17 cells, then what would be the impact. We know that T_h17 cells produce IL-17, IL-22 and IL-23 chemical messages, so the more T_h17 cells there are, then the more of these chemical messages must be floating around. A recent review (Kunkl, 2020, Feb;9(2):482) concluded that T_h17 and other T helper cells **"initiated and perpetuated an inflammatory response and the consequential neurodegeneration in MS"**. In particular, it is the increase in IL-17 and IL-22 messages that regulate cells that are resident in the central nervous system, that appear to contribute to axon (nerve fibre) damage and demyelination. Therefore, any mechanism that reduces the excess in T_h17 cells would be a sensible course of action.

Remember all this is happening in the brain and central nervous system. Therefore, the increased number of white cells have already breached the blood brain barrier.

Other Things to Consider

There is compelling evidence that T helper cells drive MS pathology, however, that is not the whole story. We have seen that increased levels of antibodies are present in the central nervous system. Therefore, the

B cells that produce them must also be present. As was noted by Jelcic et al. (Jelcic, 2018, 20 September, Volume 175, Issue 1), "**suggest that CD8^{+3} T cells, proinflammatory B cells, and autoantibodies are likely also involved. A central question is how disease-relevant T and B cells interact.**".

In fact, most of the immune-modifying medications are designed to deplete the number of B cells since high numbers of B cells were associated with more rapid disease progression.

More insidiously, B cells have been found to persist within the central nervous system of MS patients, in a layer surrounding the brain. Since some of these will be memory B cells then it has been suggested that they too may contribute to triggering a relapse or progressive loss of neurological function (Michel, 2015;6 : 636).

All of this takes place in the central nervous system. A system that is protected by the blood brain barrier. This barrier ensures that nutrients pass through to the brain, but basically blocks pathogens and large molecules. It is straight-forward to see that this barrier is compromised in MS patients. There are many papers suggesting the mechanisms that allow T and B cells to pass into the central nervous system

---

[3] CD8$^+$ are killer T cells

which I am not going to reference. For the purposes of this particular argument we know that in MS patients it is compromised.

We now have a simplified story of what goes on within the body's immune system and how the various white cells interact such that a damaging imbalance can occur. The fact is that both T and B cells cross into the central nervous system, and by interacting appear to produce excess chemical messages that appear to damage the nerve fibres.

I hope that this explanation has helped to clarify this very complex process. Please note, that I have supported the story with published research wherever possible. Now, in the best traditions of the scientific method, we should test our understanding to explore where there may be any potential gaps.

Gedankenexperiment

Einstein famously used the term, meaning 'thought experiment'. That is, where one makes a logical argument to explain what happening based on deductive or inductive reasoning. Since no actual experimentation is involved it can only ever be a hypothesis. Nevertheless, it can be a useful way of trying to build a picture of what may be happening.

The real beauty of the thought experiment is that we are not constrained with the physics of reality. We don't have to start at the beginning, we can equally well start at the end and backtrack. In this thought experiment that's what we are going to do. We shall start with damage to the myelin and work back to see if, using the information in the previous sections, we can build an understanding of what happens to someone suffering from MS.

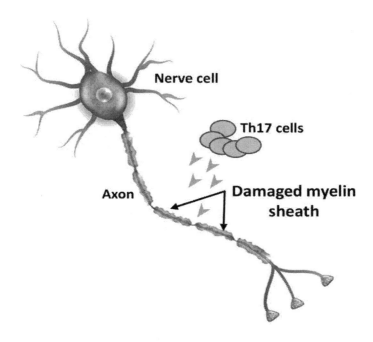

Figure 13 : Damaged Nerve by T Cell Attack

We have seen that in all likelihood the damage to the myelin is caused by the increased number of T_h17

helper cells in the central nervous system. The proportion of T_h17 cells and level of IL-17 appears to correlate with disease severity (Dos Passos, 2016, Jan 28). The number of activated T cells has explosively increased as they would to repel any invading pathogen from the few that had crossed the blood brain barrier (Fletcher, 2010, October). We also know that a cocktail of T and B cells are present in the central nervous system because the blood brain barrier has been breached from the analysis of lumber fluids.

The initiation of the attack, in all probability, started outside of the central nervous system. Some sort of trigger has started the chemical chain reaction. A reaction that ultimately leads to a plethora of primed white cells invading the central nervous system to attack the myelin sheathings.

The key question is 'what would trigger the immune system to react against the chemistry of myelin'? That key question has eluded many researchers over the years.

Recalling the ultra-low-fat regime that Swank proposed and that Jelinek has advocated, that saturated fat is bad for MS sufferers, and that its removal was a contributing factor to reducing relapses. Suppose it's not all fat, but one particular component of fat that is bad for MS? Suppose that there is a something, a protein, that triggers the immune response? One key protein in milk is suspected of molecular mimicry. That is, its structure is similar to an antigen, that it can trigger an immune response (Riccio, 2011, February 24). The molecule in question is very similar to the protein that makes up the myelin sheathing.

Introducing common sense into the discussion, one soon realises that we humans are the only mammal that drinks the milk of another. Although the majority of us have become tolerant to animal milk products over the last few thousand years, it is recognised that some still possess a weakness to milk products.

Thinking about the principles of economy, and as articulated by a medical researcher called Theodore Woodward, "when you hear hoofbeats behind you, don't expect to see a zebra", the implication being the most probable cause of the sound is a horse. The recommendation from this particular research is that MS patients should be discouraged from ingesting milk and milk products.

In our thought experiment, we could imagine that the milk protein with similar structure to the myelin sheath, could trigger an immune response in susceptible individuals. The B cell absorbs the foreign entity, presenting fragments on its surface that in turn trigger T cells. The T cells produce T_h1 and T_h17 cells.

The excess of T_h17 stimulates some white cell mechanism to attack the myelin. This could be B cells, which are instructed to multiply and produce antibodies that attack proteins on the myelin sheathing[4], or some other type of white cell such as killer T cells.

This is not far-fetched. In fact, the immune system is designed to err on the side of caution. So, if there is doubt, then it will produce a greater immune response. An extreme example of this is anaphylaxis, where the immune system overreacts as a response to an allergy and can cause the body to go into shock, like a reaction to a bee string or peanuts. In the case of MS however, the body is reacting to some stimulus, in this case, maybe a milk protein, and producing an excess of T cells.

Remember this is a thought experiment, an argument based on the knowledge that we know. As I said at the outset of this chapter, the immune system is extremely complex. Scientists and academics spend their whole lives trying to piece together an understanding of the interplays between the myriad of cells and chemical messages. The idea that this simple story will reveal all the subtleties at play is unrealistic. Nevertheless, it

---

[4] No definitive explanation has been published to date although increased numbers of B cells are measured in the central nervous system of MS patients.

helped my appreciation and understanding of some of the mechanisms that appear to be at work. Hopefully, it has been of some use to you as well.

8. The Bumpy Road

'Only those who will risk going too far can possibly find out how far one can go'. T.S. Elliot said it better that I could. Having whetted my appetite with Jelinek's approach, plus having read as much background as I could find to test the arguments, it seemed reasonable to explore other potential areas that may benefit MS sufferers. Of course, this needed to be approached with caution all the time looking for evidence. Recalling the scientific method, anyone can put forward a hypothesis, it's only with verified, repeatable evidence that it can be accepted.

On the other hand, one shouldn't be too quick to dismiss other ideas and approaches.

Ayurvedic Treatments

Ayurveda is a system of medicine from the Indian subcontinent. I liken it to Chinese medicine, of which I am extremely sceptical. Nevertheless, we were introduced to Ayurvedic treatments through a family member who had suffered from fairly severe asthma. She had seen marked improvement in her condition after attending an Ayurvedic treatment centre.

My wife arranged to travel to one of their centres in India to try one of their treatments. Since I could not find any documentation on the effectiveness or otherwise of Ayurvedic medicine, I had severe reservations of the whole process.

These reservations crystallised as I learned that the bodily substances are divided into the classical elements of earth, fire, water, air and ether. Although in Ayurveda they are combined into kapha (earth and fire), pitta (fire and water) and vata (ether and air).

Just to be clear, most Ayurvedic treatment centres seem to focus on diet, food, massage and well-being by balancing the classical elements. The treatment that I shall describe is specialised and offered by only a few clinics. However, it's the only one that I have experienced.

The central treatment offered involved a de-toxification process. The primary method is by consuming ghee (clarified butter) or a type of oil. Each day the amount of ghee or oil is increased that the patient has to consume. This goes on for a number of days until the Ayurvedic doctor feels that the patient is 'ready', by monitoring the patient's pulse. By this time the amount of ghee or oil the patient is consuming daily could be as much as 200ml. A herbal laxative is then administered, and without going into the gory details, a thoroughly miserable day is spent by the patient being cleansed.

The course also includes yoga, meditation and a strict Ayurvedic vegetarian diet. The Ayurvedic doctors also make their own medicines and prescribe these depending on the ailments they are treating.

What was most interesting was the broad section of people attending the centre and the range of ailments for which they were seeking help. There were the usual number of people looking to reduce weight. One man had prostate issues and another a heart condition. There was a lady who did have MS but was there due to the fact she had been in a car accident and needed help to improve her walking. There were some who simply wanted to attend yoga.

So, is there any conclusion? All I can give is my observation on a single case, my wife, with no scientific back up.

After the course, we returned to Scotland armed with instructions on the Ayurvedic diet and several containers of Ayurvedic medicines. We had also a good grounding in yoga as we had been practising for three hours a day for two weeks. At home we continued with the yoga as part of our exercise regime and gradually improved. My wife's balance and leg strength appeared to have improved. I cannot give a measure, but yoga positions that she could not hold when at the centre, she now can.

One other positive note was that constipation, which is common MS symptom, has disappeared. She was given Ayurvedic medicine for this, and during the course of about three months this particular symptom dissipated. Whether this was an actual effect, or whether it was coincidence there is no way to tell.

Looking at the diet we ate. It was, of course, vegetarian so devoid of any saturated animal fats. No food, with exception of fruit, is eaten raw. Most cooking is steamed. At this point it seems very healthy and aligns with Roy Swank's proposals. Any frying is done in ghee, which although a saturated fat, it does not have any milk products remaining and seems to be considered healthy in that, the consensus view, is that it doesn't produce tissue damaging free radicals.

All in all, I cannot say the experience helped my wife's MS. We learned some yoga and ate fairly healthily, which in itself cannot do any harm. My biggest concern was coming across articles that showed that some Ayurvedic medicines contained high levels of harmful substances (Breeher, 2015, October; 21(4)), such as lead and mercury.

Introduction to the Coimbra Protocol

The vitamin D story interested me. We have already discussed that vitamin D_3 is a hormone that influences a large number of processes within the body. We have also discussed how vitamin D_3 deficiency correlates with an increased occurrence of MS. In chapter 6 we saw (in a limited study) that increasing the vitamin D_3 in the blood by 10 nmol/L reduced the MS relapse rate by nearly 14%.

If we drew that as a graph it would look like the following:

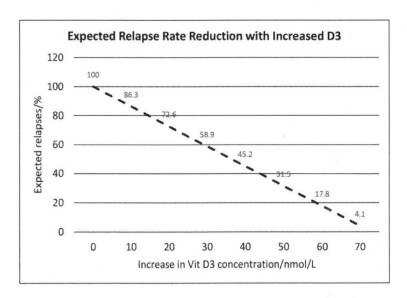

Figure 14 : Reduction in Relapses with

The question is, what is the Vitamin D_3 concentration required to eliminate relapses?

Let's assume that our MS sufferer has a vitamin D_3 concentration within the normal range, say 75 nmol/L. In order to reduce the chance of relapses to about zero we would need to increase their vitamin D_3 concentration by about 70 nmol/L to about 145 nmol/L, using the above graph to estimate the required additional dosage. This is a significant amount and well beyond what most medical practitioners would be happy to administer.

Even Professor Jelinek suggests that taking more that 10000iu/day of vitamin D_3 is ill-advised without medical supervision due to possible complications of having too much vitamin D_3 in the body. This is why we limited ourselves to 10000iu/day while I continued to search out what additional research, if any, was being undertaken. It seemed obvious that there should be a raft of work going on in this area as the story appeared to be highly compelling.

Looking for research into high dose vitamin D_3 and MS, I came across Dr. Cicero Coimbra, Department of Neurology and Neurosurgery, University of Sao Paulo. Dr. Coimbra has been administering high doses of vitamin D_3 since the early 2000s. Initially for the treatment of Parkinson's disease and then broadening his scope to treat other autoimmune disorders including MS in 2002.

In principle, in the traditions of the scientific method, the treatment builds upon existing research exploiting the link between vitamin D_3 and the multitude of cell receptors in the immune system. Large doses of vitamin D_3 are administered to increase the concentration with the blood. This helps balance the immune system, not by suppression, but by boosting the regulatory immune cells.

The Coimbra protocol of high dose vitamin D_3 is dependent on the specifics of the patient and therefore needs to be conducted under medical supervision. Not only, to get the dosage levels correct, but also to monitor the impact of very high doses on the body. High levels of vitamin D_3 could lead to too much calcium in the body which could impact the kidneys.

I'm not going to explain the whole treatment as it's more complex that simply vitamin D_3. What I was most interested in was the claimed successes. Basically, the claim is that the protocol can successfully suppress MS activity in about 95% of cases! If that's true, then that's an astounding figure. Remember the prescribed drug my wife was taking (Tecfidera) has a claimed benefit of reducing relapses in about 60% of patients. Not suppressing the disease, only reducing the probability of a relapse.

Dr. Coimbra and his team claim to have treated more than 4000 patients with the protocol in his Sao Paulo clinic. The reason I use the word 'claim', is not that I doubt him, but I have no other evidence to confirm the numbers. I would find it extraordinary for a whole team to manufacture numbers, so I am reasonably convinced that the figures are genuine. Dr. Coimbra has also trained a number of medical professionals around the world, and I'm sure that if they thought there was little merit in the protocol then they would not waste their time on it.

I was very keen to ensure that whoever we contacted would have a bona fide medical background and was working in a hospital. Fortunately, there is a published list of trained medics on the 'This is MS' bulletin board. Interestingly, there were no Coimbra trained professionals in the UK (2017). We selected our doctor and after some email exchanges made our way to Italy for an appointment.

It was February 2017 when we had our first appointment. The protocol was fully explained, the breadth and number of tests that my wife would have to have to ensure that the treatment was effectively managed. The greatest benefit of physically meeting the treatment doctor is a very human one. It's when you look into their eyes and gauge whether they are simply 'pill pushing' or whether they feel the treatment is something they believe in and is worth pursuing. I have to say, that after our session, I was supremely optimistic in the Coimbra method. Of course, there are no guarantees. There are no guarantees in anything in life apart from death and taxes. However, based on the arguments that had led us to this appointment and our doctor's confidence that the protocol had benefits, based on her own experience. We signed up.

The Treatments

The treatment itself is very straight-forward. Large quantities of vitamin D_3 are taken orally. The typically starting dose is estimated at about 1000iu/kg/day, together with a cocktail of additional vitamins and magnesium tablets. Due to large vitamin D_3 dose there are some restrictions in diet that must be followed to keep calcium intake low, whilst maintaining very good hydration. Interestingly, in order to minimise calcium intake, dairy products have to be avoided. If molecular mimicry is a factor, then fortuitously this protocol removes this particular risk.

The important thing is to have a complete chemical analysis after a couple of months to ensure that there are no undesired effects. Then blood and urine chemistry are regularly checked every few months and the vitamin D_3 dose adjusted if required. I'm not going to go into detail here as it is fully documented elsewhere and in the Coimbra protocol itself.

It is not possible to directly evaluate the impact of the increased levels of vitamin D_3 on the immune system. So, it is necessary to track the quantity of PTH (parathyroid hormone) in the blood. Basically, vitamin D_3 will suppress the amount of PTH in the blood. Each individual is different, hence the need to tailor the amount of vitamin D_3 the patient requires. The ideal dose of vitamin D_3 is when the PTH measure is at its lowest normal limit. It is key that this is monitored by a medical professional.

That really is it. Keep the PTH at a nominal level and eventually the body should be protected from any relapses or degradation.

The dilemma that I faced, if you like, was the lack of hard statistical data of cause and effect of the Coimbra protocol. That is, except for the claim that it had successfully halted progression and in a large number of cases, and had resulted in some improvements in other cases.

I think that we have hit on a fundamental problem when dealing with people. It's all very well doing lots of experiments on mice and having models that represent humans to try and build up a picture of understanding. This is the general process that neurologists and pharmacologists follow, and necessarily have to prove, before human trials are allowed. However, suppose someone had a procedure that could halt the progression of some disease with a success rate of 95%. And suppose that they wished to carry out a trial with volunteers that would take some considerable time, say more than 10 years. And suppose when assembling the volunteers, it was mentioned that half of them would be in the placebo group, then I think a very human response would be not to bother to take their chances with the unproven method and remain with their existing medication.

So, based on the Coimbra claims and the fact that our trained medical professional had a great deal of confidence in the method, I put my natural scepticism to one side.

Our Actual Journey

Following our consultation, my wife started with the high dose vitamin D_3 in March 2017. I think my problem was and is impatience. I knew that it would take time, but as they say, 'hope springs eternal'.

My wife diligently followed the protocol, in particular ensuring that she kept herself well hydrated. The diet was easily followed since we had been following Jelinek's diet which is slightly more restrictive. I knew that it would take significant time to show any results, if any, so we maintained our life as normal, and the protocol just became a minor consideration each day.

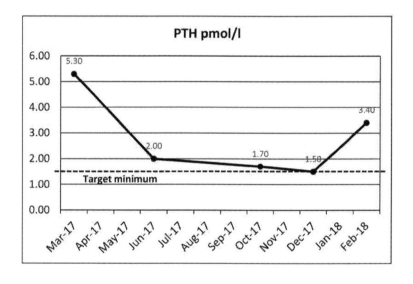

Figure 15 : PTH Measure 2017-18

I have included my wife's PTH measures for the first year. All went well for the first few months, but towards the end of the year the PTH increased as her body resisted the vitamin D_3. At this point she was effectively out of treatment, although I have to point out that there was no material change that I could detect.

Following a consultation, the vitamin D_3 dose was significantly increased and we continued with the process.

Throughout the second year all appeared to be going well. By the time we reached January 2019 (two years on the protocol) I felt that my wife's walking was gradually improving. It's totally a subjective impression, but one of our favourite restaurants is about 1.5km from the house. Historically, my wife would feel her legs very heavy after about 1km and it would be an effort to complete the journey. Now, there seemed to be a renewed strength. Of course, it was not perfect, but she seemed to be managing the 1.5km walk with an increased level of confidence. I was pleasantly optimistic.

However, events conspired against us.

As I said before my wife had been prescribed Tecfidera by our local neurologist. I was concerned, not only by its reported impact, but also the fact that I could not find out how it works except for the fact that it did seem to suppress white blood cells (Khatri, 2015, Jul;4(4)). After some discussion we decided that my wife would stop talking the Tecfidera, thus making the Coimbra protocol the only ongoing treatment.

We're not sure what went wrong, whether there was a bounce from removing the Tecfidera from the equation, but whatever it was my wife's PTH level crashed.

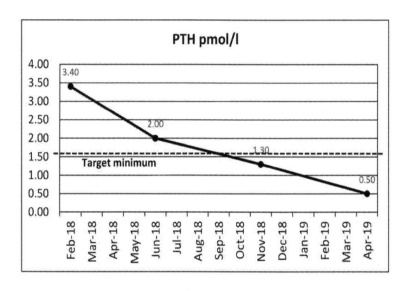

Figure 16 : PTH Measure 2018-19

Hypercalcemia

In March 2019, the first signs started to appear. They were not obvious, at least not to anyone not explicitly looking for them. My wife gradually became weaker.

Walking a few hundred meters became an effort. My first fear was that it was a relapse, but we couldn't detect any new symptoms that are usually, but not always, associated with a relapse. There were also additional signs like stale breath, confusion and heart palpations. I began to suspect hypercalcemia, but were waiting on our regular test results which had been delayed due to some re-organisational issues at the pathology laboratory.

Fortuitously, my wife had had a blood test at our local doctor, who phoned us immediately and had my wife admitted to hospital. It was indeed hypercalcemia. There was too much vitamin D_3 in her blood which was resulting in an excess of calcium in her blood which was now having an impact on her kidneys.

It took a few days to stabilise her condition and all vitamin D_3 therapy was suspended.

This is the key danger with this treatment and one that we were trying to be very careful to avoid. We had not changed anything in our life apart from stopping the Tecfidera. Although all the advice suggested that there should be no linkage between vitamin D_3 therapy and Tecfidera, that was the only change we made. That was my thinking at the time. However, in retrospect, when you examine the gradient of the PTH curve it was clear that the downward trajectory had been consistent for some time. Therefore, blaming the hypercalcemia as a consequence of stopping Tecfidera seems unjustifiable.

It is interesting to note that Jelinek's approach recommends continuing with any prescribed medication. Clearly, we did not do that. This, I believe, was a mistake. Not that it would have impacted the downward trajectory of PTH, but it would have given my wife some protection against MS once we halted the vitamin D_3 protocol.

I think the learning point is not simply monitoring the value of the PTH, but watching the rate of change and as it nears the desired minimum value, and increasing the frequency of the blood and urine tests. If we had done that, then we would have probably identified the falling PTH before it became critical.

Reviewing the Protocol

As I said before too much vitamin D_3 is dangerous. That's why fat-soluble additives should only be taken under medical supervision.

As we have seen from the previous diagrams, it takes a long time for vitamin D_3 to build up in the body. The evidence being how long it took to supress the PTH measure. Similarly, it takes a very long time for the body to break down the vitamin D₃.

One of the key threats of an excess of vitamin D, apart from hypercalcemia, is the effect on kidney function. Therefore, during the following months whilst the vitamin D₃ therapy was suspended, regular monitoring of kidney function ensued.

The typical reference values for creatinine for women is in the range 45-90 μmol/L. During the following year we monitored the level at regular intervals and restarted the vitamin D₃ therapy, albeit at the reduced dose of 5000iu/day. The logic being to offer some basic protection.

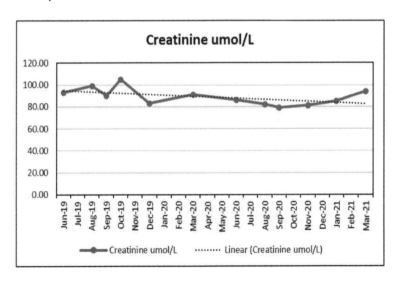

Figure 17: Tracking Kidney Function

The creatinine levels, although still on the high side are not too concerning, we have been advised. Nevertheless, we shall not resume full treatment until our medical practitioner is confident that no damage can occur.

The painful truth is that all medication carries a risk. Even the humble aspirin is not without risk. For example, it should not be given to children recovering from flu or chickenpox for fear of Reye's syndrome. A rare, potentially fatal condition, that impacts the brain and liver.

So, we are at a juncture. A waiting game, while my wife's chemistry stabilizes, while we weigh up the risks and potential benefits, or do nothing. It's not in my nature to do nothing and having the sense of improvement prior to the hypercalcemia incident (hoping that it was not a placebo effect), it seems that we shall restart the protocol when we can. In the meantime, we continue with the Jelinek approach which we had been following anyway. That is, a low-fat diet, no dairy and regular exercise.

The sense of frustration at starting again, however, is palpable.

9. Improving Behaviour

So far, we've discussed the journey my wife and I have been on with her MS. To be specific, it's been her journey. Now it's time for us to assess the journey that I, as her partner, have been on, and how that has impacted our relationship.

To be honest, I have found this section the most difficult to write as it's completely subjective but requires a certain objectivity on my part. In addition, I'm not good at self-criticism, particularly when I believe that I have a goal of improving the status quo.

With this admission in mind, I have tried to document my character flaws and the areas of annoyance and frustration that I have brought to the journey.

Twenty Questions

I said at the outset that I was originally trained as a scientist. There are good things and bad things with such a training. On the good side, there is an enquiring mind, a thirst for knowledge and the need to understand on a fundamental level how things work. On the bad side, when it comes to a relationship, there is an enquiring mind, a thirst for knowledge and the need to understand on a fundamental level how things work. Yes, it's a double-edged sword.

The problem with being a partner in this journey is that the only information that one receives is via observation and then questioning. It's just a traditional science experiment. Unfortunately, in this case the subject is my wife.

As we discussed in the scientific method, any hypothesis can only be accepted once it has been supported by observational evidence. Therefore, observation is the foundation of establishing fact. This resulted in behaviour modification on my part. I watched for changes, any mis-step, any foot dragging, any sign of instability. If I detected something, anything that was out of the ordinary, then I followed it up with a question. 'How are you feeling; are you alright; how is the strength in your legs?' This was the mantra. In my mind this was the only way to confirm or contradict what I perceived. However, from my wife's point of view the questioning, which started as an irritation, became an increasing annoyance. A focus that was a constant reminder that all was not well and an insidious attack on her independence.

Invariably my questions were met with heavy sighs and occasionally a stare that would have put Medusa to shame. This was often followed by a lecture about how the 'twenty questions' made her feel and that sometimes she dreaded being out with me.

I am not going to say that I successfully modified my behaviour. I have tried, but my training is deeply ingrained and therefore difficult to dramatically alter. This is an ongoing battle that I'm trying to deal with, and one that I suspect that the partners of other MS sufferers will also have to be aware of and have to manage.

Cognition

I am very fortunate that I seem to have a good memory. Not only carrying fairly useful information, but also an inordinate amount of trivia. The upshot of this is that I tend to remember dates, appointments, bills, to-do lists and social engagements. I also have pretty good recall at details within stories.

It is well known that MS often impacts cognition. So much so, that my wife does have periodic tests as part of her ongoing care within the health system. The good news is that to date there has been no measured degradation in her acuity.

Nevertheless, I do find myself 'helping out' when she is looking for an answer to something or other, or when relating a story. This is another annoying trait that I have developed, and something that I need to actively guard against.

I have tried to reason why there appears to be no measurable reduction in cognition, yet my very unscientific perception is that her acuity is less than it used to be. My only conclusion is that she has gradually become over dependent on the use of her diary, which she adopted some time ago out of a fear of forgetting things. This, now, may have become a crutch that makes one's memory lazy.

Although I try to stop myself auto-correcting, I do encourage my wife to continue to exercise her mind, either writing a diary or playing Scrabble and other games.

Don't Make Assumptions

There is an old saying about assuming something, that it makes an 'Ass' out of 'U' and 'Me'. Apart from being very trite, there is an element of truth in the saying. In particular, assuming something about someone else is not only extremely annoying it belittles that person in their mind. So much so, that the person may start to doubt their own abilities.

It's like I said in the previous section about 'helping out' too much. Assuming that someone cannot do something or being over cautious can sap the very confidence that it is necessary to build.

Of course, it's a balance. It's necessary to be there for support and encouragement and to ensure that your partner is not putting themselves into an unnecessary risk situation, whilst giving them the freedom to live their life. I know this sounds obvious, but it was, and probably still is, one of the great pit-falls into which I tend to fall

The judgement of balance is tricky. However, one begins to learn after a number of heated discussions and fights. Allow the person to ask for help if needed. Not to be callous, but the occasional knock is probably worth it in the long term, if the patient is to build their confidence and in so doing their self-esteem.

Patience

They say patience is a virtue, and for very good reason. Of all my failures, patience is right up there in neon lights. As you may have perceived from reading the previous chapters that once I have a goal, then I am fairly driven to try and achieve it, and to achieve it as quickly and efficiently as possible.

This character trait can be useful in many types of business. However, when dealing with one's nearest and dearest, the lack of patience is extremely counter-productive.

After my wife's initial diagnosis, we were both struggling through the early stages of the SARA curve. The idea that we had any sort of normal future seemed quite remote. However, following the discovery of Jelinek and then Coimbra, my optimism received a kick start, and as a consequence my impatience at a lack of measurable progress increased.

Provided one can shield the MS patient from the partner's overt impatience and frustration, then all should be relatively fine. Unfortunately, my wife knows me too well, and could see the stress that I was self-inflicting. This came to a head following the hypercalcemia episode.

As I said earlier, after almost two years following the Coimbra protocol, I felt that my wife was making good progress when we had the incident. Everything had to stop and it was eight long months before we could re-start the treatment (with the reduced dose). Maybe someone who is fundamentally more patient than I would have handled it better, but my sense of wasted time and effort weighed heavily upon me.

This was perhaps a chance to grow as a person. Dusting ourselves down and having to start again, perhaps with a more realistic appreciation of what is or is not possible and the required timeframes. I did feel it was essential to keep positive about the treatments we had been following and to keep my wife enthused.

So, all in all, I am trying to improve my patience. There is no panacea. Given what I've learned and what we have experienced, I feel there are some approaches and treatments that can help. What is clear, is that a lot of patience is required.

Tactful Risk Management

One of the more difficult roles that the partner has to play is one of risk manager. It is a delicate balance of trying to maintain the life that we had with a new reality. This, whilst maintaining patience, and trying to allow the MS sufferer as much independence as realistically possible.

It was most apparent with our holidays. We had always liked to travel. Not just sitting on a beach, but also exploring some of the far-flung parts of the world. We even enjoyed city breaks, which had always involved exploring, mainly on foot.

MS changes all that. It's no longer possible to walk miles through the back streets of Paris or Prague sampling local cuisine and culture. No longer is it possible to undertake cycling trips. Also, care must be taken when booking somewhere exotic that the temperatures are not too high due to heat intolerance.

I was always the one who booked our holidays, and therefore, I had the role of risk manager. I had to be cognisant of the potential dangers and the necessary mitigations that we needed to adopt. I also had to do this in as tactful way as possible and to be as supportive as possible.

Fortunately, with a few minor adjustments it is possible to maintain the desired lifestyle.

City breaks can continue, and by using the various city tour 'hop on-hop off' buses, has meant that we can still enjoy the local culture.

Cycling, unfortunately to date, has not been possible. Although we are exploring the possibility of accessing electrical assisted three-wheel cycles.

Unfortunately, tours to interesting sites become more expensive, since group tours can, in general, only manage everyone moving at the same pace. Therefore, it is necessary to make private arrangements and use a lot more taxis. Again, it's not difficult, it's just something for which one has to recognise and prepare.

The most useful invention in recent years, in my opinion, is that of the trolley bag, the four wheeled variety. My wife travels with this at all times. It gives her the stability and confidence that she needs, so much so, she frequently outpaces me when in an airport.

Of course, it's not just holidays or activities. Although I am keen for the day when my wife can take up some form of cycling, her priorities are somewhat different. She used to have a sizable shoe collection. All sorts, but certainly an impressive array of high heel shoes. As her stability became impaired it became necessary to make the move to flatter shoes. This was done gradually and reluctantly. On the plus side, she does have a number of nieces who are extremely pleased with their acquisitions.

Very high heels are, in my opinion, risky at the best of times, but with reduced stability they should definitely be avoided. My wife's goal is to one day be able to re-master walking in heels. Not the highest, but at least with some sort of heel.

Although not ideal, as I have illustrated, there are measures that can be taken to make life more 'normal'. These adjustments can only be achieved with open and honest communication, and any decisions made, must be made jointly.

Having a career that includes a lot of project and programme management, risk mitigation is one of my strengths. I believe that this is where a partner can offer the significant support by leading the difficult discussions and being suitably empathetic. Of course, in my case, all my frailties outlined in the foregoing sections still need to be addressed.

Not Rock Hudson, James Bond

In the introduction I mentioned a melodrama starring Rock Hudson where he cured his blind girlfriend. I want to re-emphasise that I'm not Rock Hudson in so many ways. I am also completely realistic that I'm not going to suddenly discover a cure for MS that has been eluding the professional scientific community. However, I do feel that there is a lot of really good information available to give us clues that we can use to improve the life of MS sufferers. A lot of which I have tried to outline in the previous chapters.

The point I'm trying to make is that, as a partner to someone with MS, we are all capable of helping improve their lives. Whether it's researching as much as possible to be able to challenge the treatments that are prescribed, and thus empowering the MS sufferer to be in control of their therapy. Alternatively, becoming more empathetic and listening to their daily experiences may provide enough support and encouragement to make them feel just that little bit better.

The bottom line is that we, partners, all need to exhibit the qualities of patience, empathy, the ability to listen and not to endlessly over question. We all need to do this, and I suspect that I need to do it more than most!

I recall a time management course that I went on years ago. They were trying to promote the idea of organising one's whole life. The key thing was that regardless how bad your day had been, before you went home for the evening, one needed to take a deep breath and reflect upon who your partner wished to see when you walk through the door. Is it the guy who has issues with the world or someone smooth, sophisticated and in control? Who will it be, the cantankerous boor or James Bond? Each of us needs to strive to be 007.

10. Final Discussion

At this point you are probably expecting me to write that all is well. My wife has completely recovered and we are leading an exciting and normal life. I'm afraid that I shall have to disappoint you. Life is not perfect and as you will have read in the previous chapters, we have faced our issues with which we are still having to tackle.

However, I am going to use this chapter as a recap of the key points and to discuss some of the evidence that I have presented, and to work out what the next course of action, for us, should be.

Root Cause

We saw in the early chapters the definite link between diet and MS relapse rate. We also saw that the amount of sunshine seemed to have a major impact on the occurrence of MS. We learned that vitamin D_3 appeared to reduce the number of relapses, and the fact that a significant number of MS sufferers appear to have lower than normal vitamin D levels.

If MS had a simple single cause, then in all probability there would have been more progress at addressing the condition over the past few decades than has happened. Clearly, by definition, multiple sclerosis is multiple attacks, with no single mechanism. Therefore, establishing a single root cause has always been elusive.

I have a great deal of sympathy for the medical and bioscience community. The mechanisms at play are extremely complex. The messages, message sequencing and feedback loops between the cells of the immune system make the understanding of what's going on very difficult to fathom. I recall a joke involving a physicist:

> A farmer has problem with his chickens not laying. He approaches a physicist to help.
> The physicist says he can help, but the solution will only work for a spherical egg in a vacuum.

The point is that when dealing with people the conditions are far from ideal. People are not uniform entities. They are variable, possess behavioural differences, and cannot be controlled like a laboratory experiment. Any tests and trials require large scale statistical sample populations in order to determine the influencing factors. Even then, results can often be interpreted subjectively.

The greater the number of variables or degrees of freedom in any experiment requires larger sample populations which can be difficult to arrange. Therefore, caution must be exercised when interpreting the results of experiments with small sample populations.

Remembering our thought experiment, we know that the myelin around the nerves is being destroyed in all probability by a process driven by T_h17 helper cells. Therefore, we know the immune system is out of balance. The reason that it gets out of balance is difficult to isolate. It could be genetic, it could be infection induced, or it could be something in the environment. A single root cause seems unlikely.

However, we have seen evidence of how diet can influence relapse rates, in particular how the removal of saturated fats can improve the long-term health of MS sufferers. We have also seen that sunshine, that is living somewhere sunny, reduces the likelihood of developing MS. Artificially increasing the vitamin D_3 level in place of producing it naturally from sunlight also reduces relapse rate, and we understand how this helps to balance the proinflammatory T_h17 cells that are generally thought to be a key driver of MS.

We have discussed also what may be a likely trigger for the disease by the body reacting to proteins that are similar in nature to myelin. So called molecular mimicry.

Common sense would suggest, based on the information we have discussed, that low vitamin D possibly due to environmental or hereditary reasons, and an immune response triggered possibly by molecular mimicry may drive MS. Undoubtably, the mechanisms and interactions within the immune system are complex and making such a sweeping statement based on limited evidence is dangerous. Nevertheless, there is wealth of data out there and using it does suggest some obvious courses of action.

Remembering our discussion on the scientific method, it is worth recalling Occam's razor. An idea attributed to a Franciscan monk, William of Ockham, that when presented with competing hypotheses that make the same predictions, one should select the solution with the fewest assumptions. Paraphrasing, this becomes 'the simplest solution is most likely the right one'. Now, I am not suggesting that there is a simple solution to halting MS progression, however, there does seem to be significant evidence that vitamin D may help to rebalance the immune responses. If that is indeed to case, then that may be a key treatment. Reduced fat intake will help reduce risk factors as was shown by Swank (R.L. Swank, 1990). I guess the question, which I cannot answer, is whether it's all saturated fats or one or more particular fats that may be triggering a response?

Now What?

The key question is for us to determine our next steps. As you will have gathered, I am very keen on making any decision based on scientific evidence. The problem with such a complex multi-faceted disease, together with the huge body of research work available, some of which can appear to be contradictory in nature, is that it can be difficult to build a picture of what is actually happening.

During the vitamin D treatment, we hit a bump. As I described, this has necessitated us stopping the treatment while my wife's body rebalances itself. However, since we felt that she was making good progress, we fully intend re-starting the protocol, under medical guidance, when appropriate.

This may be a reset. Restarting from the beginning, which is rather frustrating in the sense of wasted time. Nevertheless, the choice of following a fairly benign treatment of managing one's diet, taking exercise and vitamin D, or taking a cocktail of immunosuppressant or immune-modifiers. The choice for us is straightforward.

I am not for an instant discounting the work that is going on in the scientific community. Should there be a 'miracle cure' suddenly announced, then I shall be very interested. So, I do keep my eye, as we all should, on the current research. So much so, that I was encouraged to read that a team in Boston identified a subset of T_h17 cells that were extremely damaging to myelin. These cells could then be targeted by gene therapy (Hou, 2019 Oct 8;116(41)). Of course, it's early days, but it's good to know that, perhaps, progress is being made.

My current battle is disappointment and impatience, having seen progress, albeit slight, and then having to stop our chosen path, at least temporarily. However, as we know there is no cure for MS, so in good time we should be able to restart. I suppose the up-side is that we are lucky enough to have the time.

Being a Better Partner

In the last chapter I openly discussed my weaknesses. Needless to say, I am trying to work on them. I think the biggest message is not to treat one's partner as an invalid. The patient is grown-up and mature and perfectly capable of asking for help if and when they need it. The need to continually ask 'how are you', is a reflection of the partner's anxiety.

Unfortunately, I am human and was trained as a scientist. The need for constant questioning is heavily ingrained. I see this as my uphill challenge. Although writing this text has been cathartic and has given me the focus to try to address these weaknesses.

For all other partners out there supporting an MS patient, please learn from my mistakes.

Finally

I hope this journey hasn't been too onerous and may be of some help to those of you who are facing the uphill battle with MS. I have shown that there is a body of evidence to help you evaluate whatever course of treatment you have adopted. I also hope that I have stressed the importance of ensuring that there is always factual evidence available, and not to be taken in by the peddling of 'snake oil', which is still prevalent whenever fear and desperation set in.

I hope that I have shown that there is no need for dogma and that it's alright to change one's view provided the facts support it. As the economist John Maynard Keyes is reported to have said, "when my information changes, I alter my conclusions. What do you do, sir?"[5]

I started this chapter expressing my disappointment that my wife's MS was not a thing of the past. It is my fervent hope that I shall be able to update this text in few years' time with a more complete story, ideally with a better ending. In the meantime, we shall continue with our journey based on all the information that I have gathered, together.

---

[5] No direct evidence has been found that Keynes made this comment.

References

Anderson, T. (1972, Sep 23 107(6)). Vitamin C and the common cold: a double-blind trial. *Canadian Mediacl Journal*, 503-508.

Angell, M. (2005). *The Truth about the Drug Companies: How They Deceive Us and What to Do about It.* Random House Inc; Reprint edition (9 Aug. 2005).

Baquet, L. e. (2018;6:e6037). Short-term interval aerobic exercise training does not improve memory functio in relapsing-remitting multiple sclerosis - a randomised controlled trial. *PeerJ*.

Borst, P. (2008 Dec 2; 105(48)). Mega-dose vitamin C as therapy for human cancer? *Proceedings of the National Academy of Sciences USA*.

Breeher, L. (2015, October; 21(4)). A cluster of lead poisoning among consumers of Ayurvedic medicine. *Int J Occup Environ Health*, 303-307.

Cantorna, M. (2015 Apr 7(4)). Vitamin D and 1,25(OH)2D Regulation of T cells. *Nutrients*, 3011-3021.

Chang, S. (2010, December 10). Vitamin D Suppresses Th17 Cytokine Production by Inducing C/EBP

Homologous Protein (CHOP) Expression. *Journal Biological Chemistry*, 38751-38755.

Damsker, J. (2010, January:1183). Th1 and Th17 cells Adversaries and collaborators. *Annals of the New York Academy of Sciences*, 211-221.

Dankers, W. e. (2019; 10:1504). Human Memory Th17 Cell Populations Change Into Anti-inflammatory Cells With Regulatory Capacity Upon Exposure to Active Vitamin D. *Frontiers in Immunology*.

Deisenhammer, F. (2019, Apr 12). The Cerebrospinal Fluid in Multiple Sclerosis. *Frontiers in Immunology*.

Dos Passos, G. S. (2016, Jan 28). Th17 Cells Pathways in Multiple Sclerosis and Neuromyelitis Optica Spectrum Disorders: Pathophysiological and Therapeutic Implications. *Mediators of Inflammation*.

Esparza M.L., S. S. (1995; 142(7)). Nutrition, latitude, and multiple sclerosis mortality: an ecologic study. *American Journal of Epidemiol*, 733-737.

Fletcher, J. L. (2010, October). T cells in multiple sclerosis and experimental autoimmune encephalomyelitis. *Clinical and Experimantal Immunology*, 162(1):1-11.

Gornall, J. (2016, July 4). How I Beat MS. *Daily Mail*. Daily Mail.

Hadgkiss, E. J. (2015). The association of diet with quality of life, disability, and relapse rate in an international sample of people with multiple sclerosis. *Nutritional Neuroscience, April*, 125-136.

Halabchi, F. A. (2017; 17:185). Exercise prescription for patients with multiple sclerosis; potential benefits and practical recommmendations. *BMC Neurology*.

Hewison, M. (2010, June:39(2)). Vitamin D and the immune system: new perspectives on an old theme. *Endocrinol Metab Clin North Am*, 365-379.

Hou, L. e. (2019 Oct 8;116(41)). SerpinB1 controls encephalitogenic T helper cells in neuroinflammation. *Procedings National Academy of Science USA*.

Jelcic, I. e. (2018, 20 September, Volume 175, Issue 1). Memory B Cells Activate Brain-Homing, Autoreactive CD4+ T Cells in Multiple Sclerosis. *Cell*, 85-100.

Jelinek, G. (2016). *Overcoming Multiple Sclerosis*. London: Allen & Unwin.

Jinlu Ji, H. Z. (2019, 23 Mar). The role and mechanism of vitamin D-mediated regulation of Treg/Th17 balance in recurrent pregnancy loss. *American Journal of Reproductive Immunology*.

Karagkouni, A. (2013, Aug;12(10)). Effect of Stress on Brain Inflammation and Multiple Sclerosis. *Autoimmune Review*, 947-53.

Khatri, B. (2015, Jul;4(4)). The effect of dimethyl fumarate (Tecfidera™) on lymphocyte counts: A potential contributor to progressive multifocal leukoencephalopathy risk. *Multiple Sclerosis Related Disorders*, 377-379.

Kimball, S. (2007 Sep;86(3)). Safety of vitamin D3 in adults with multiple sclerosis. *American Journal of Clinical Nutrition*, 645-51.

Kubler-Ross, E. (1969). *On Death and Dying.* New York: Macmillan.

Kunkl, M. (2020, Feb;9(2):482). T Helper Cells: The Modulators of Inflammation in Multiple Sclerosis. *Cells*.

Lee, G. (2018, Mar; 19(3)). The Balance of Th17 versus Treg Cells in Autoimmunity. *International Journal of Molecular Sciences*.

Malkiewicz, M. e. (2019; 16:15). Blood-brain barrier permeability and physical exercise. *Jounal Neuroinflammation*.

Malosse, D. P. (1992; 11(4-6)). Correlation between milk and dairy product consumption and multiple sclerosis prevalence: a worldwide study. *Neuroepidemiology*, 304-12.

Michel, L.-O. (2015;6 : 636). B Cells in the Multiple Sclerosis Central Nervous System: Trafficking and Contribution to CNS-Compartmentalized Inflammation. *Frontiers in Immunology*.

Mokry, L. e. (Aug 25, 2015). Vitamin D and Risk of Multiple Sclerosis: A Mendelian Randomization Study. *PLOS Medicine*.

Munger, K. e. (2006 Dec 20;296(23)). Serum 25-hydroxyvitamin D levels and risk of multiple sclerosis. *Journal of the American Medical Association*, 2832-8.

Nagelkerken, L. (January 1998). Role of Th1 and Th2 cells in autoimmune demyelinating disease. *Braz J Med Biol Res*, Vol 31(1) 55-60.

Nistala, K. W. (2009, Volume 48, Issue 6). Th17 and regulatory T cells: rebalancing pro- and anti-inflammatory forces in autoimmune arthritis. *Rheumatology*, 602-606.

Pauling, L. (1976). *Vitamin C, the Common Cold and the Flu.* San Francisco: W H Freeman.

Pennock, N. (2013 Dec; 37(4)). T cell responses: naïve to memory and everything in between. *Advances in Physiology Education*, 273-283.

Pierot-Deseilligny, C.-P. P. (2012 5(4)). Relationship between 25-OH-D serum level and relapse rate in multipl sclerosis patients before and after viatamin D supplementation. *Therapeutic Advances in Neurological Disorders*, 187-198.

Pilz, S. e. (2018, Jul 17). Rationale and Plan for Vitamin D Food Fortification: A Review and Guidance Paper. *Frontiers in Endocrinology.*

R.L. Swank, B. D. (1990, July 7). Effect of low saturated fat diet in early and late cases of multiple sclerosis. *The Lancet*, 37-39.

Read, C. (1898). *Logic Deductive and Inductive.* London: Pantiano Classics.

Riccio, P. (2011, February 24). May Diet and Dietary Supplements Improve the Wellness of Multiple Sclerosis Patients? A Molecular Approach. *Autoimmune Diseases.*

Russell, W. (1976). *Multiple Sclerosis : Control of the Disease.* Oxford: Pergamon Press.

Senders, A. L. (2012; 2012:567324). Mind-Body Medicine fo Multiple Sclerosis: A Systematic Review. *Autoimmune Diseases.*

Shirani, A., & al., e. (2012;308(3)). Association between use of interferon beta and progression of disability in patients with relapsing-remitting multiple sclerosis. *JAMA*, 247-256.

Swingler, R. C. (1986;49). The distribution of multiple sclerosis in the Uniteed Kingdom. *Journal of Neurology, Neorosurgery and Psychiatry*, 1115-1124.

Tremlett, H. (2008 Apr 14(3)). Natural history of secondary-progressive multiple sclerosis . *Multiple Sclerosis Journal; Pub Med.*, 314-24.

von Geldern, G. (2012 : 8). The influence of nutritional factors on the prognosis of multiple sclerosis. *Nature Reviews Neurology*, 678-689.

Weber, M. H. (2011, February, Volume 1812, Issue 2). The role of antibodies in multiple sclerosis. *Molecular Basis of Disease*, 239-245.

Williams, R. (1956). *Biochemical Individuality: The Basis for the Genetotrophic Concept* . John Wiley & Sons.

Yada, V. M. (2015). Low-fat, plant based diet in multiple sclerosis : A randomized controlled trial. *Multiple Sclerosis and Related Disorders 9*, 80-90.

Zhang, X. W. (2014, Sept., Vol. 8, No. 5). Role of Vitamin D3 in Regulation of T Helper Cell 17 and Regulatory T-Cell Balance in Rats With Immunoglobulin A Nephropathy . *Iranian Journal of Kidney Diseases*.

About the Author

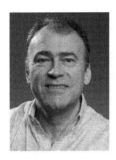

Garry Alexander was educated in Applied Physics at the University of Strathclyde in Glasgow, Scotland. Following which he studied for a Ph.D. in the dynamics of ship motions to improve their stability in extreme conditions. He then pursued a career in telecommunications and software development. Finally, being involved in data quality and management for a multi-national business, and authoring a book on the subject.

Over the past few years, he has become more involved with climate science with a view to reducing individuals' carbon footprints.

This book was a personal project to empower MS sufferers with as much information as could be contained in a concise volume, with the aim of helping those starting upon the journey.

Manufactured by Amazon.ca
Bolton, ON

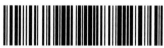